Top 60 signs for nurses:
QUICK REFERENCE GUIDE FOR BEST PRACTICE CARE

Top 60 signs for nurses:
QUICK REFERENCE GUIDE FOR BEST PRACTICE CARE

Mark Dennis MBBS (Honours), FRACP
Cardiologist, Intensive Care Trainee
Royal Prince Alfred Hospital
Camperdown, NSW, Australia

William Talbot Bowen MBBS, MD, FAAEM
Board Certified Emergency Medicine Physician
Lompoc Valley Medical Center
Lompoc, CA, United States

Lucy Cho BA, MBBS, MIPH
Medical Officer
Kirketon Road Centre
Kings Cross, Sydney, NSW, Australia

ELSEVIER

ELSEVIER

Elsevier Australia. ACN 001 002 357
(a division of Reed International Books Australia Pty Ltd)
Tower 1, 475 Victoria Avenue, Chatswood, NSW 2067

Notice

This publication has been carefully reviewed and checked to ensure that the content is as accurate and current as possible at time of publication. We would recommend, however, that the reader verify any procedures, treatments, drug dosages or legal content described in this book. Neither the author, the contributors, nor the publisher assume any liability for injury and/or damage to persons or property arising from any error in or omission from this publication.

National Library of Australia Cataloguing-in-Publication entry

Dennis, Mark, 1978- author.
Top 60 signs for nurses : quick reference guide for best practice care / Mark Dennis, William Talbot Bowen, Lucy Cho.
9780729542388 (paperback)
Includes index.
Nursing diagnosis—Handbooks, manuals, etc.
Symptoms—Handbooks, manuals, etc.
Diagnosis—Handbooks, manuals, etc.
Bowen, William Talbot, author.
Cho, Lucy, author.

Senior Content Strategist: Larissa Norrie
Content Development Specialist: Lauren Santos
Senior Project Manager: Karthikeyan Murthy
Edited by Katie Millar
Proofread by Annabel Adair
Illustrations by Toppan Best-set Premedia Limited and Alan Laver
Design by Natalie Bowra
Index by Robert Swanson
Typeset by Toppan Best-set Premedia Limited
Printed by 1010 Printing International Ltd.

Contents

Preface

When we started the voyage of writing a textbook based on clinical medicine and clinical signs we hoped it would be valued by clinicians. We have been heartened by the response of the readership and their feedback. It is clear from this that nursing clinicians have a similar but different focus to our physician readers. Whilst the main text of *Mechanisms of Clinical Signs* is robust, it may not be practical for the fast-paced busy wards that nurses practise in. Moreover, a more focused handbook would allow for easier reference in the time-pressured environment.

Therefore, we have developed *Top 60 signs for nurses: Quick reference guide for best practice care*. Requested and reviewed by junior and senior nursing staff alike, this title is focused on the requirements of the nursing fraternity. Only selected signs recommended by reviewers have been included, making it more accessible and more relevant to the specific needs of the nursing staff.

Acknowledgements

The authors would like to thank their families and friends for their unwavering support; it takes a village. Finally, to all the medical students who continue to ask 'why' and who have, with more senior clinician guidance, provided direction for improvements of the text – thank you.

60 signs reviewers list

All chapters

Carmen Axisa RN BN MClinN (Cardiothoracic) PhD (candidate)
Lecturer, Faculty of Health, University of Technology Sydney

Jane Currie MSc BSc(Hons)
Lecturer/Nurse Practitioner, University of Sydney, Sydney Nursing School, NSW, Australia

Matthew Barton BMedSc(Hons) MN PhD
Lecturer Griffith University, Queensland, Australia; Research Fellow, Menzies Health Institute, Queensland, Australia

Jacqueline Bloomfield PhD MN PGDip (Healthcare ED) PGDip (Midwifery) BN RN
Associate Professor, Sydney Nursing School, The University of Sydney, NSW, Australia

Trish Burton DipAppSc BSc BAppSc MEd PhD FACN
Senior Lecturer, Nursing, College of Health and Biomedicine, Victoria University, Victoria, Australia

Assoc Professor Helen Forbes RN PhD
Associate Head of School, School of Nursing and Midwifery, Deakin University, Geelong, Australia

Amy Johnston BSc(Hons) BN GradDipAdEd MEd PhD
Research fellow, Gold Coast Health and Menzies Health Institute, Queensland, Australia

Janice Layh RN RM Mst Adv Nursing Prac PhD Candidate
University of The Sunshine Coast, Queensland, Australia

Nancy McNamara PhD Candidate MHSc BN RN CATE
Senior Academic Staff Member, Wintec, New Zealand

Judith Needham EdD MN BN RN RM
Senior Lecturer – Director of Professional Practice, School of Nursing and Midwifery Griffith University, Queensland, Australia

Jane Truscott PhD MBA MS
Nurse Practitioner, Aspen Medical and Senior Lecturer, Central Queensland University, Queensland, Australia

Elizabeth Watt RN RM MNS FCNA
Lecturer, School of Nursing and Midwifery, La Trobe University, Bundoora, Victoria, Australia

Reviewers

Chapter 1 Respiratory Signs:
Dr Keith Wong MBBS(Hons) MMed(Clin Epi) PhD FRACP
Research Fellow, Sleep and Circadian Research Group, Woolcock Institute of Medical
Research; Staff Specialist, Department of Respiratory and Sleep Medicine, Royal Prince
Alfred Hospital, University of Sydney

Professor Ivan Young PhD FRACP
Clinical Professor, Central Clinical School (Medicine), University of Sydney;
Department of Respiratory Medicine, Royal Prince Alfred Hospital

Chapter 2 Cardiovascular Signs:
Dr Rajesh Puranik MBBS PhD FRACP
Consultant Cardiologist, Royal Prince Alfred Hospital, NHMRC/NHF Postdoctoral
Fellow, University of Sydney

Chapter 3 Haematological and Oncological Signs:
Professor Douglas Joshua MD
Professor of Internal Medicine, University of Sydney; Head of Institute of Haematology,
Royal Prince Alfred Hospital

Chapter 4 Neurological Signs:
Dr John Carmody MB BCh MRCPI FRACP
Staff Specialist Neurologist, Hon. Clinical Senior Lecturer, University of Wollongong

Associate Professor Leo Davies MD MB BS FRACP
Sub-Dean and Head of Assessment, Sydney Medical School, University of Sydney;
Australian & New Zealand Association of Neurologists; Australian Association of
Neurologists

Chapter 5 Gastroenterological Signs:
Associate Professor Meng C Ngu MBBS(Hons) BMedSc(Hons) PhD FRACP
Clinical Associate Professor, University of Sydney; Consultant Gastroenterologist

Chapter 6 Endocrinological Signs:
Professor Stephen Twigg MBBS (Hons-I) PhD FRACP
Professor in Medicine, Central Clinical School and the Bosch Institute, University of
Sydney; Senior Staff Specialist in Endocrinology, Royal Prince Alfred Hospital

Awais Saleem Babri MBBS, PGDipSc, PhD, GradCertEdu
School of Biomedical Sciences, The University of Queensland, Qld, Australia

Timothy Billington PhD
Lecturer Medical Sciences and Medical Education, School of Medicine, University of
Wollongong, NSW, Australia

Wai Ping (Alicia) Chan MBBS FRACP PhD FCSANX

Abbreviations

ADP	adenosine diphosphate	JVP	jugular venous pressure
ADH	antidiuretic hormone, or vasopressin	LA	left atrial
		LPS	lipopolysaccharides
ARDS	acute respiratory distress syndrome	LR	likelihood ratio
		LV	left ventricular
ASD	atrial septal defect	MRI	magnetic resonance imaging
AV (node)	atrioventricular (node)		
AVM	arteriovenous malformation	NPV	negative predictive value
		OSA	obstructive sleep apnoea
CGRP	calcitonin gene-related peptide	PCWP	pulmonary capillary wedge pressure
CHF	congestive heart failure	PDA	patent ductus arteriosus
CI	confidence interval	PDGF	platelet-derived growth factor
cMOAT	canalicular multispecific organic anion transporter	PFO	patent foramen ovale
CMV	cytomegalovirus	PGI_2	prostaglandin I_2
COPD	chronic obstructive pulmonary disease	PICA	posterior inferior cerebellar artery
CNS	central nervous system	PLR	positive likelihood ratio
CRAO	central retinal artery occlusion	PND	paroxysmal nocturnal dyspnoea
CSA	central sleep apnoea	PPV	positive predictive value
CSF	cerebrospinal fluid	PTH	parathyroid hormone
CVP	central venous pressure	RA	right atrial
DI	diabetes insipidus	RAA(S)	renin–angiotensin–aldosterone (system)
ENAC	epithelial sodium (Na) channel	RAR	rapidly adapting receptor
HIV	human immunodeficiency virus	RTA	renal tubule acidosis
		T_3	triiodothyronine (thyroid hormone)
HLA	human leukocyte antigen		
HOCM	hypertrophic obstructive cardiomyopathy	TB	tuberculosis
		V2 (receptor)	arginine vasopressin receptor 2
HPOA	hypertrophic pulmonary osteoarthropathy		
		VEGF	vascular endothelial growth factor
HSV	herpes simplex virus		
IVC	inferior vena cava	vWF	von Willebrand factor

CHAPTER 1

RESPIRATORY SIGNS

Accessory muscle breathing

Respiratory system revisited

Apart from the lungs, the respiratory system is made up of three main components: the central control centre, sensors and effectors.

The brainstem contains several centres in the pons and medulla, which (in addition to other parts of the brain) regulate inspiration and expiration. It receives information from a variety of receptors that monitor the partial pressure of oxygen and carbon dioxide as well the stretch and compliance of the lung and irritants in the lung and upper airways. The central control system sends messages via nerve fibres such as the phrenic nerve to control respiratory rate and depth of breathing, in response to the data it receives.

Damage, disruption or alterations to any of these three – brainstem, nerves, receptors – can cause specific signs.

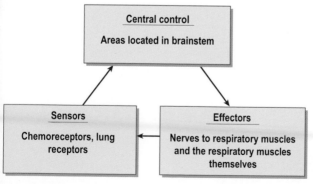

FIGURE 1.1
Simplified respiratory control
Based on West JB, West's Respiratory Physiology, *7th edn, Philadelphia: Lippincott Williams & Wilkins, 2005: Fig 8-1.*

CLINICAL PEARL

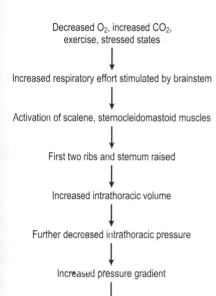

Decreased O_2, increased CO_2, exercise, stressed states

↓

Increased respiratory effort stimulated by brainstem

↓

Activation of scalene, sternocleidomastoid muscles

↓

First two ribs and sternum raised

↓

Increased intrathoracic volume

↓

Further decreased intrathoracic pressure

↓

Increased pressure gradient

↓

Greater volume inspired

FIGURE 1.2
Physiology behind accessory muscle respiration

Description

Normal inspiration involves only the diaphragm. Expiration occurs passively due to elastic recoil of the lungs. When inspiratory effort requires the use of the sternocleidomastoid, scalene, trapezius, internal intercostal and abdominal muscles, the 'accessory muscles' of breathing are said to be in use.

Condition/s associated with

Any state resulting in an increased effort of breathing:

- Chronic obstructive pulmonary disease (COPD)
- Asthma
- Pneumonia
- Pneumothorax
- Pulmonary embolism
- Congestive heart failure (CHF)

Mechanism/s

In times of increased respiratory effort, the accessory muscles of breathing are invoked to exaggerate the normal respiratory process. Use of the accessory muscles can create more negative intrathoracic pressure on inspiration (pulling more air in and possibly causing *tracheal tug*) and more positive pressure on expiration (pushing air out).

On inspiration, the scalene and sternocleidomastoid muscles help lift and expand the chest wall, allowing for a decrease in intrathoracic pressure and increased air entry.

On expiration, the abdominal muscles help push air out of the lungs.

Sign value

The use of accessory muscles is a non-specific finding but is valuable in assessing the severity of respiratory difficulty (i.e. the 'work' of breathing). More than 90% of acute exacerbations of COPD present with accessory muscle use.[1] One study showed a sensitivity of 39% and specificity of 89% with a PLR of 4.75.[2] In children, accessory muscle use is a clear sign of increased respiratory effort.

Agonal respiration

Description
Slow inspirations with irregular pauses. Patients are often described as gasping for air. Agonal breathing is usually closely followed by death unless intervention is provided.

Condition/s associated with
Any aetiology leading to imminent death.

Mechanism/s
Agonal respiration is thought to be a brainstem reflex, providing a last-ditch respiratory effort for the body to try to save itself. It is thought of as the last respiratory effort before terminal apnoea.[3]

Sign value
Without intervention, agonal respiration heralds impending death. Studies have shown that recognition of agonal breathing may improve recognition of cardiac arrest,[4] and implementation of protocols designed to identify agonal breathing over the phone can significantly increase the diagnosis of cardiac arrest by emergency dispatchers.[5] It is absolutely a sign that must be managed without delay.

Apnoea

Description
A pause in breathing.

Condition/s associated with

Central sleep apnoea (CSA)

- Brainstem injuries – stroke, encephalitis, cervical trauma
- Congestive heart failure (CHF)
- Opiates
- Obesity-related hypoventilation syndrome (Pickwickian syndrome)

Obstructive sleep apnoea (OSA)

- Obesity
- Micrognathia
- Alcohol
- Adenotonsillar hypertrophy

Mechanism/s
Apnoeas can be classified into central or obstructive, depending on the location of the causal pathology.

Central sleep apnoea
In central apnoeas, a lack of *respiratory drive* from the respiratory centre causes a break in breathing. There is a complex array of factors contributing to this form of apnoea.

- Injury to the brainstem ventilatory/respiratory centres (see Figure 1.1) – which normally regulate breathing – can cause diminished, inconsistent or absent respiratory drive.

- Opiate drugs, working via the *mu* receptors in the brainstem, decrease the central drive to breathe, even though the required networks remain intact.

- In obesity hypoventilation syndrome, it is thought that the body cannot compensate for the obstructed respiratory mechanics. This, combined with blunted chemoreceptor sensitivity, causes apnoea – although the mechanism is not clear.[6]

- Patients with motor neuron disease, myasthenia gravis, polio and other neurodegenerative diseases have a central respiratory drive but this drive does *not get transmitted* to the respiratory muscles to enable effective ventilation.

- *Cheyne–Stokes breathing* is a form of central sleep apnoea and is discussed in Chapter 2, 'Cardiovascular signs'.

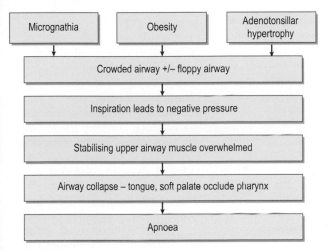

FIGURE 1.3
OSA mechanism

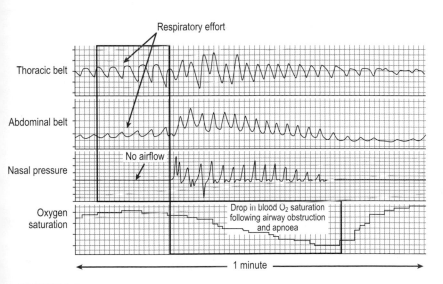

FIGURE 1.4
Polysomnogram of obstructive sleep apnoea in a patient with heart failure

Khayat R et al. Sleep-disordered breathing in heart failure: identifying and treating an important but often unrecognized comorbidity in heart failure patients. Journal of Cardiac Failure *2013; 19(6): Fig 4.*

Obstructive sleep apnoea

The negative pressure of inspiration leads to collapse of the airway, causing a temporary obstruction or occlusion of the nasopharynx and oropharynx. Most commonly, the tongue and palate move into opposition with the posterior pharyngeal wall, causing obstruction of the airway.[7]

Anything that crowds or destabilises the airway (e.g. micrognathia, adenotonsillar hypertrophy, obesity or acromegaly) may contribute to collapse and obstruction.

Alcohol can relax the normal stabilising muscles of the pharynx.

Obstructive apnoeas can be witnessed but can also be detected on polysomnography.

Sign value

Obstructive apnoea is an important clinical sign. There is substantial evidence that persistent apnoeas during sleep adversely affect glucose control and blood pressure management as well as increasing the risk of stroke, coronary artery disease and heart failure, among many other complications. Obstructive apnoeas reduce sleep quality, and increase daytime somnolence and irritability. They should be suspected if these symptoms are described in context.

Central sleep apnoeas are often manifestations of underlying diseases and must be monitored for. They are always pathological and if present may require intervention.

Asymmetrical chest expansion

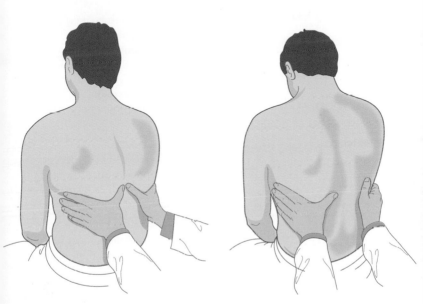

FIGURE 1.5
Palpation to detect asymmetry of chest expansion, a sign of pleural effusion

Diaz-Guzman E, Budev MM. Accuracy of the physical examination in evaluating pleural effusion. Cleveland Clinic Journal of Medicine *2008; 75(4): 297–303.*

Description

The clinician is positioned behind the patient, usually looking down at the clavicles (upper lobe movement) or palpating the chest wall (lower lobes). As the patient breathes, uneven extension of the chest wall in inspiration or retraction on expiration may be observed. This may manifest itself as an absolute difference or a slight lag in expansion.

Condition/s associated with

More common

- Pneumonia
- Pleural effusion
- Flail chest
- Foreign body
- Pneumothorax

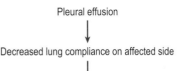

Pleural effusion

↓

Decreased lung compliance on affected side

↓

Decreased expansion on inspiration relative to normal side

FIGURE 1.6
Mechanism of pneumonia

Less common

- Unilateral diaphragm paralysis
- Haemothorax
- Musculoskeletal abnormality (e.g. kyphoscoliosis)
- Neuropathy
- Pulmonary fibrosis – localised

Mechanism/s

Symmetrical bilateral expansion of the chest wall is reliant on normal musculature, nerve function and lung compliance. Therefore, any abnormality unilaterally affecting a nerve, muscle or the compliance of the lungs may produce an asymmetrical expansion.

Pneumonia, pleural effusions

If pneumonia (consolidation of the airways) and/or pleural effusions (fluid in the pleural space) are present, the normal compliance of the lung is reduced. When inspiration occurs, the affected lung will have decreased expansion compared to normal.

Foreign body

In the lung blocked by a foreign body, air cannot get past the larger airways to the small airways to allow normal expansion.

Flail segment

A flail chest or flail segment is usually caused by trauma. Sections of ribs become detached from the chest wall. As the segment is no longer attached to the expanding chest on inspiration, it is susceptible to negative

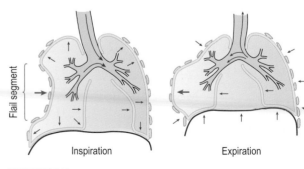

FIGURE 1.7
Flail segment mechanism

Based on Aggarwal R, Hunter A. BMJ. http://archive.student.bmj.com/issues/07/02/education/52.php [28 Feb 2011].

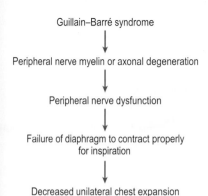

Guillain–Barré syndrome

↓

Peripheral nerve myelin or axonal degeneration

↓

Peripheral nerve dysfunction

↓

Failure of diaphragm to contract properly
for inspiration

↓

Decreased unilateral chest expansion

FIGURE 1.8
Mechanism of unilateral chest expansion

intrathoracic pressure. This pressure sucks the flail segment inwards on inspiration and pushes it out on expiration (opposite to the intact remaining chest wall).

Kyphoscoliosis

Progressive forward and/or lateral curvature of the spine (kyphoscoliosis) may become so severe that it mechanically depresses one lung over the other and causes decreased chest expansion on one side.

Unilateral diaphragm paralysis

If unilateral diaphragmatic paralysis occurs for any reason, the side of the affected diaphragm will not contract, affecting lung expansion.

Sign value

Asymmetrical chest expansion is always pathological. While there have been very few studies, asymmetrical chest expansion was shown to be one of the most effective signs in predicting the presence of a pleural effusion, ahead of vocal resonance and vocal fremitus. It was an independent predictor of pleural effusion[8] with an odds ratio of 5.22, sensitivity of 74% and specificity of 91%.

Barrel chest

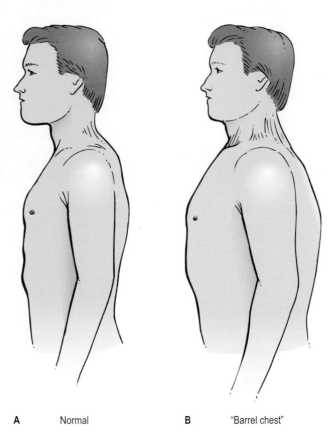

A   Normal   **B**   "Barrel chest"

FIGURE 1.9
Barrel chest

Swartz MH, Textbook of Physical Diagnosis: History and Examination, *6th edn, St Louis: Mosby, 2004.*

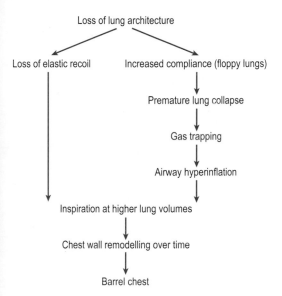

FIGURE 1.10
Mechanism of barrel chest in emphysema

Description

A ratio of anteroposterior (AP) to lateral chest diameter of greater than 0.9. The normal AP diameter should be less than the lateral diameter and the ratio of AP to lateral should lie between 0.70 and 0.75.

Condition/s associated with

- Chronic bronchitis
- Emphysema

Also occurs in elderly people without disease.

Mechanism/s

Considered to be due to over-activity of the scalene and sternocleidomastoid muscles, which lift the upper ribs and sternum.[9] With time, this overuse causes remodelling of the chest.

In chronic obstructive pulmonary disease, there is a chronic airflow limitation that results in increased end-expiratory volumes and chronic hyperinflation.

Chronic hyperinflation reduces airway resistance and improves elastic recoil at the expense of higher lung volumes. Over time this leads to chest wall remodelling and barrel chest abnormality.[10]

Bradypnoea

Description

An unusually slow rate of breathing, usually defined in an adult as less than 8–12 breaths per minute.

Condition/s associated with

Bradypnoea may occur in any condition or state that affects the respiratory/ventilatory centres of the brain or brainstem.

More common

- Drugs – opiates, benzodiazepines, barbiturates, anaesthetic agents
- Respiratory failure
- Brain injury and raised intracranial pressure
- Hypothyroidism
- Excess alcohol consumption

Less common

- Hypothermia
- Uraemia
- Metabolic alkalosis

Mechanism/s

Bradypnoea can be caused by:

- decreased central nervous system output – i.e. a defect or reduction in central respiratory drive that diminishes messages 'telling' the body to breathe (e.g. brain injury, raised ICP, opiate overdose)
- disorders in the nerves connecting to the respiratory muscles (e.g. motor neuron disease)
- disorders of the muscles associated with breathing (e.g. muscle tiredness in respiratory failure)
- respiratory compensation in response to a metabolic process (e.g. in response to metabolic alkalosis, the body will reduce respiration in an attempt to retain carbon dioxide and acids).

Sign value

Although not specific, bradypnoea in an unwell patient is often a sign of serious dysfunction and requires immediate attention. In asthma and respiratory failure, bradypnoea often precedes respiratory arrest.

Breath sounds: vesicular or normal

Description

Vesicular or normal breath sounds can be heard over the lung fields and are low pitched and soft. The inspiratory portion of the sound is longer than the expiratory and there is no pause between these phases.

Vesicular breath sounds can be conceptualised and contrasted with bronchial breath sounds. Figure 1.11 shows that vesicular breath sounds have a longer inspiratory limb and bronchial breath sounds a more prominent expiratory phase.

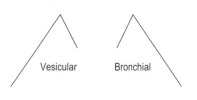

Vesicular   Bronchial

(c) 2006, Kanchan Ganda, M.D.

FIGURE 1.11
Differences between vesicular and bronchial breath sounds

http://ocw.tufts.edu/Content/24/lecturenotes/311144/312054_medium.jpg

Condition/s associated with

• Normal lung fields

Mechanisms

Lung sounds are produced by vertical and turbulent flow.[11]

Several studies[12,13] have suggested that the inspiratory portion of the vesicular breath sound is *regionally* produced by turbulence in the lobar, segmental and smaller peripheral airways, while expiratory elements of vesicular breath sounds are attributed to flow through the larger airways. Contrary to popular belief, vesicular breath sounds are NOT produced by air entering the vesicles or alveoli.[14]

Vesicular breath sounds are transmitted sounds from the airways which are *muffled or filtered* by air-filled alveoli, so only lower frequencies are transmitted. Low frequencies are not well heard by the human ear and therefore seem softer than bronchial breath sounds.

Sign value

Vesicular breath sounds provide the baseline with which to compare other sounds and their recognition is therefore essential in identifying and understanding abnormalities.

Breath sounds: bronchial

Description

Loud, harsh, high-pitched breath sounds that are normal if heard over the tracheobronchial tree but abnormal if heard over lung tissue on auscultation. As opposed to vesicular breath sounds, the expiratory portion of the cycle is longer and there is often a pause between inspiration and expiration.

Condition/s associated with

- Normal over trachea
- Pneumonia
- Pleural effusion – heard above the actual effusion
- Adjacent to large pericardial effusion
- Atelectasis
- Tension pneumothorax

Mechanism/s

As previously explained under 'Breath Sounds', bronchial breath sounds are not normally heard over the lung fields, as the chest wall and alveoli muffle higher-frequency sounds. In the presence of consolidation, however, the alveolar 'filter' is replaced by a medium (such as pus) that transmits sound (and higher frequencies), better[15] allowing bronchial breath sounds to be heard.

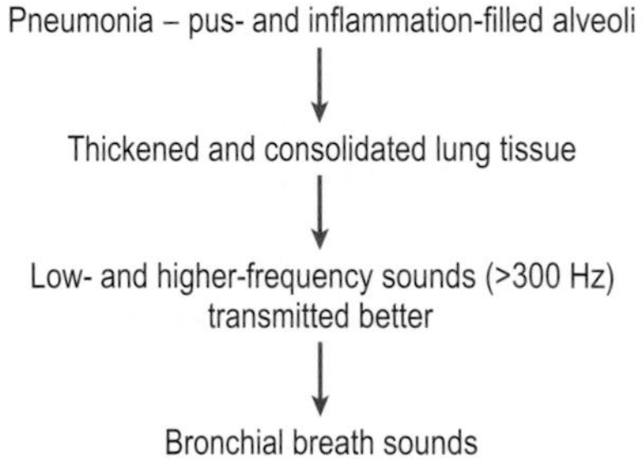

Pneumonia – pus- and inflammation-filled alveoli

↓

Thickened and consolidated lung tissue

↓

Low- and higher-frequency sounds (>300 Hz) transmitted better

↓

Bronchial breath sounds

FIGURE 1.12
Mechanism of bronchial breath sounds

Atelectasis/collapse mechanism/s

Bronchial breath sounds can also be heard in the presence of alveolar collapse or atelectasis. In these conditions the alveoli are compressed by fluid (e.g. pleural fluid) or have collapsed owing to poor inspiration (e.g. being bed bound or pain restricting breathing). Collapsed alveoli also act as an effective transmitter of sound and higher frequencies.

Sign value

In patients with cough and fever, bronchial breath sounds suggest pneumonia (sensitivity 14, specificity 96%, LR 3.3)[9] and are a valuable sign.

Breath sounds: reduced or diminished

Description

Low-intensity, soft breath sounds (compared to vesicular).

Condition/s associated with:

- Emphysema/chronic obstructive pulmonary disease
- Pleural effusion

- Low flow states – elderly patients, poor inspiration
- Low transmission states – muscular or obese body habitus

Mechanism/s

Breath sounds are related to the intensity of *flow (sound energy)* as well as the *transmission* of the sounds through the lungs and chest wall.

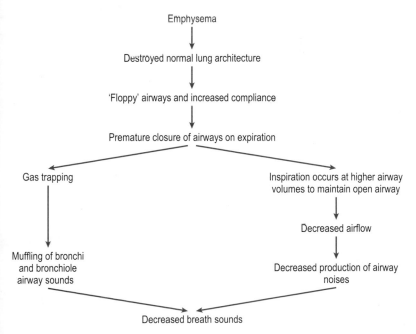

FIGURE 1.13
Mechanisms of decreased breath sounds in emphysema

Pneumonia/consolidation – bronchial breath sounds or diminished breath sounds?

Consolidation with pus, as happens with pneumonia, has been described as producing diminished and bronchial breath sounds.

How is this possible?

If the consolidation *blocks off airways* that are also surrounded by consolidation, then there will be no flow and no sound (i.e. decreased breath sounds).

If the underlying airways are *patent* and surrounded by consolidated material, then bronchial breathing is heard.

Thus it is the patency of the airways which determines what is heard.

Abnormalities of either element will diminish breath sounds.

Emphysema/chronic obstructive pulmonary disease mechanism/s

Decreased transmission of breath sounds due to airway destruction and increased gas trapping creating muffling of noise is thought to contribute to the diminished breath sounds present in COPD.[16] However, some research has suggested decreased production of airway noises due to decreased airflow may be the predominant cause.[17]

Low flow states

The production of vesicular breath sounds is dependent on flow. This is influenced by respiratory effort. In patients with poor respiratory effort due to any cause (e.g. drug-induced respiratory depression, age and frailty, neuromuscular disease), flow rates will be lower and therefore breath sounds softer. In cases of foreign body obstruction, there is no flow past the blockage and therefore no sound is generated.

Low transmission states

Even if airflow is normal, the transmission of lung sounds can be impeded by pulmonary or extra-pulmonary factors.[14]

Obesity is one example of an extrapulmonary impedance. Excess adipose tissue prevents the normal transmission of lung sounds during auscultation. Within the chest, the presence of gas (pneumothorax) or fluid (pleural fluid) between the airways and stethoscope may also reduce transmission.[14]

Sign value

Breath sounds have been extensively researched and have variable value depending on clinical context. Table 1.1 summarises a selection of studies reviewing altered breath sounds. Like all signs, they need to be interpreted in the light of presentation and augmented with appropriate additional tests.

More recent studies are now looking at the use of computerised lung sound analysis to improve specificities of the sounds traditionally heard via stethoscope. Initial reviews suggest this technology may be of value.[18]

Breath sound score/intensity – a more objective assessment

The breath sound score developed by Pardee[19] is a more systematic approach to identifying and scoring breath sounds The clinician assesses by.

1. Listening to the chest in six locations
   » bilateral upper anterior chest
   » bilateral midaxillae
   » bilateral posterior bases
2. Scoring each site for inspiratory sounds

   0 – absent
   1 – barely audible
   2 – faint but definitely heard
   3 – normal
   4 – loud

3. Adding up the points

A very low score is specific but not sensitive for chronic obstructive lung disease, and a very high score significantly decreases the likelihood of chronic obstructive lung disease being present.

TABLE 1.1
Breath sounds and vocal resonance*

Finding (reference)[+]	Sensitivity (%)	Specificity (%)	Likelihood ratio[+] if finding is	
			Present	Absent
Breath sound score				
Detecting chronic airflow obstruction[15,20]				
≤9	23–46	96–97	**10.2**	–
10–12	34–63	–	**3.6**	–
13–15	11–16	–	NS	–
≥16	3–10	33–34	**0.1**	–
Diminished breath sounds				
Detecting pleural effusion in hospitalised patients	88	83	**5.2**	**0.1**
Detecting chronic airflow obstruction[21–24]	29–82	63–96	**3.2**	0.5
Detecting underlying pleural effusion in mechanically ventilated patient[25]	42	90	**4.3**	0.6
Detecting asthma during methacholine challenge testing[26]	78	81	**4.2**	**0.3**
Detecting pneumonia in patients with cough and fever[27–30]	15–49	73–95	2.3	0.8

TABLE 1.1
Breath sounds and vocal resonance—cont'd

Finding (reference)[†]	Sensitivity (%)	Specificity (%)	Likelihood ratio[‡] if finding is	
			Present	Absent
Asymmetrical breath sounds after intubation				
Detecting right main-stem bronchus intubation[31,32]	28–41	98–99	**24.4**	0.7
Bronchial breath sounds				
Detecting pneumonia in patients with cough and fever[27]	14	96	**3.3**	NS

*Diagnostic standard: For chronic airflow obstruction, FEV_1 <40% predicted (breath sound score) or FEV_1/FVC (%) ratio <0.6 to 0.7 (diminished breath sounds); for underlying pleural effusion, chest radiography or (if mechanically ventilated) computed tomography; for asthma, FEV_1 decreases ≥20% during methacholine challenge; for pneumonia, infiltrate on chest radiograph; for right main-stem intubation, chest radiograph[31] or direct endoscopic visualisation.[32]

†Definition of findings: For breath sound score, see text; for diminished vocal resonance intensity, the transmitted sounds from the patient's voice when reciting numbers, as detected by a stethoscope on the patient's posterior chest, are reduced or absent.

‡Likelihood ratio (LR) if finding present = positive LR; LR if finding absent = negative LR.

NS, not significant.

McGee S, Evidence Based Physical Diagnosis, 3rd edn, St Louis: Elsevier, 2012: EBM Box 28-1.

Crackles (rales)

Description

Non-continuous, explosive popping sounds heard more often on inspiration but which can also be present on expiration. Crackles may be described as fine or coarse. Coarse crackles are associated with the larger airways and fine crackles with smaller branches.

Inspiratory crackles[14]

- Normally present in dependent lung areas
- Not transmitted to mouth
- Not influenced by cough
- May be influenced by gravity, posture
- Shorter duration – 5 msec, higher frequency

Expiratory crackles

- Late inspiration/expiration
- Heard throughout lung, transmitted to mouth
- Can change or disappear on coughing
- Longer duration – 15 msec, lower frequency

Condition/s associated with

There are many causes of crackles, the common ones being:

- asthma
- COPD
- bronchiectasis
- pulmonary oedema/congestive heart failure
- pneumonia
- lung cancer
- interstitial lung disease (pulmonary fibrosis).

Common causes of crackles and their features are summarised in Table 1.2.

Mechanism/s

In all types of crackles, either altered architecture of the lung parenchyma (e.g. from pulmonary fibrosis) and/or the accumulation of secretions with accompanying inflammation or oedema causes the airways to narrow, obstruct or collapse.

Inspiratory crackles (more common) occur when the negative pressure of inspiration causes airways that have previously collapsed to 'pop' open.[33] Once open, there is a sudden equalisation of pressure on either side of the obstruction, resulting in vibrations of the airway wall, creating the sound.

Expiratory crackles are more controversial in terms of their mechanism. Two theories have been proposed:

1. The 'trapped gas hypothesis' suggests that there are areas of airway collapse and that the positive pressure of expiration forces these open, causing crackles as they burst apart.

TABLE 1.2
Characteristics of common crackles

Pulmonary fibrosis	Short duration crackles, mid to late inspiratory fine crackles[34]
Bronchiectasis	Coarse, early to mid inspiratory[35]
COPD	Scanty, early, low pitched, ending before mid-point of inspiration.[35] End-point is later than crackles in bronchiectasis
Heart failure	Late inspiratory crackles,[36] quickly resolve with appropriate treatment
Pneumonia	Mid inspiratory, coarse, similar to bronchiectasis in acute period.[35] During recovery, end inspiratory and short, similar to pulmonary fibrosis[37]
Sarcoidosis	Fine, mid to late inspiratory – fewer in nature than pulmonary fibrosis and differing locations

2 Recent studies have shown that expiratory crackles are more likely to be due to sudden collapse or closure of some areas on expiration[33] (i.e. the pressures needed to keep small airways open are not maintained when breathing out and so these smaller areas collapse).

Bronchiectactic crackle mechanism/s

The destruction of elastic and muscular components of the bronchi walls that occurs in bronchiectasis can cause the bronchi to collapse on end expiration. The sudden opening at inspiration is thought to generate the crackle.[35]

COPD crackle mechanism/s

The most common cause of crackles in COPD are probably airway secretions.[35] Continuous crackles throughout inspiration and expiration have been described and are attributed to the opening and closing of bronchi, due to destruction of normal lung parenchyma and support structures.[35]

Pneumonia crackle mechanism/s

Pneumonia may present with crackles in two ways:

1 Acutely – owing to infiltration of inflammatory cells, pus and oedema which fill or narrow the airways. Inspiration may abruptly open these blocked airways and generate sound.

2 Later – in the resolving stage of illness it is thought that oedema decreases but inflammatory cells are still present. The lung becomes drier, leading to reduced compliance in some parts, causing segmental airway collapse.[35]

Sign value

A very valuable sign.

Even if heard with normal breathing, crackles are most likely pathological. Various types of crackles have been shown to be associated with different pathologies:

- Fine, late inspiratory crackles and pulmonary fibrosis: sensitivity 81%, specificity 86%, positive likelihood ratio (PLR) 5.9.[21] These fine crackles can be heard BEFORE the development of radiological abnormalities in pulmonary fibrosis patients,[38] making them very valuable in identifying early disease and monitoring for drug toxicity (e.g. amiodarone lung fibrosis).

- Coarse or fine, late or pan-inspiratory crackles and elevated left atrial pressure in patients with a cardiomyopathy and congestive heart failure: PLR 3.4.[22]

- Early inspiratory crackles and chronic airflow obstruction: specificity 97–98%, PLR 14.6[22] and in detecting severe disease in patients with chronic airflow obstruction: sensitivity 90%, specificity 96% and, if present, PLR 20.8.[39]

- Auscultation has been found to be as accurate as CT in identifying areas of asbestosis lung disease and may have a role in non-invasive screening.[14,22,40]

Expiratory crackles are a lot less common, especially in COPD, are not specific and are present in many other lung complaints.

The reduction of crackle duration may have potential as an outcome measure for respiratory therapy intervention.[41] Similarly, advanced computerised techniques to assess respiratory sounds have shown promise in objective diagnosis[42,43] and outcome following intervention.[44]

Dyspnoea

Description

Strictly a symptom and not a sign, dyspnoea is the subjective awareness that an increased amount of effort is required for breathing.

Condition/s associated with

- Anxiety
- Respiratory disorders – COPD, pulmonary fibrosis, pneumonia
- Cardiac disorders – heart failure
- Anaemia
- Bronchoconstriction
- Deconditioning

General mechanism/s

The mechanism of dyspnoea is complex, involving many parts of the respiratory control system (summarised in Figure 1.14). Causes can be broadly grouped by:

1. conditions in which central respiratory drive is increased ('air hunger')
2. conditions where there is an increased respiratory load ('increased work of breathing') or
3. conditions where there is lung irritation ('chest tightness', 'constriction').[23,24]

Keeping these three groups in mind will help make the common pathways easier to understand.

Common pathways

Mechanical loading, respiratory effort and 'corollary discharge'

At times of increased respiratory load or effort, there is a conscious awareness of the activation of the muscles needed to breathe. This sense of effort arises from the brainstem and increases whenever the brainstem signals to increase muscle effort, when the breathing load increases or when muscles are weakened, fatigued or paralysed.[23,24]

In other words, when the CNS voluntarily sends a signal to the respiratory muscles to increase the work of breathing, it also sends a copy to the sensory cortex telling it there is an increased work of breathing. This phenomenon is called 'corollary discharge'.[23]

Chemoreceptors

It has been shown that hypercapnia makes an independent contribution to the experience of breathlessness.[25,26] It is thought that hypercapnia may directly be sensed as 'air hunger', regardless of ventilatory drive.

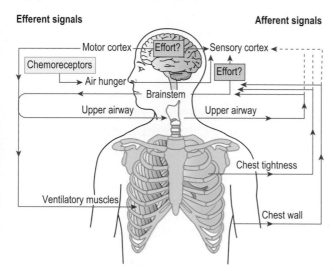

FIGURE 1.14
Mechanisms involved in the sensation of dyspnoea
Based on Manning HL, Schwartzstein RM, N Engl J Med *1995; 333(23): 1547–1553.*

Chemoreceptors: which, what and where?

Peripheral chemoreceptors
- Located in carotid and aortic bodies
- Respond to pO_2, increased pCO_2 and H^+ ions

Central chemoreceptors
- Located in medulla
- Sensitive to pCO_2 **not** pO_2
- Respond to changes in pH of cerebrospinal fluid (CSF)

Hypercapnia also leads to increased brainstem ventilatory output or drive (to blow off the excess carbon dioxide) and this leads to a corollary discharge (as explained above).

Hypoxaemia also contributes to increased ventilation and respiratory discomfort, although it plays a lesser role than hypercapnia. It is unclear whether hypoxaemia causes dyspnoea directly or via increasing ventilation that is then sensed as dyspnoea.

Mechanoreceptors

- *Upper airway receptors.* The face and upper airway have receptors (many of which are innervated by the trigeminal nerve) that can modulate dyspnoea. Mechanoreceptors in the upper airway have been shown to excite or inhibit expiratory and inspiratory muscles and modulate the intensity of dyspnoea.[23]

- *Pulmonary receptors.* The lung has three types of receptors (slowly adapting receptors, rapidly adapting receptors (RARs) and C-fibres) that transmit information back to the brainstem and brain about airway tension, lung volume and the state of the lung. These receptors can be stimulated by mechanical or chemical influences. Information detected is transmitted by the vagus nerve (CNX) back to the CNS, where, depending on the stimulus, it can be perceived as irritation, chest tightness, air hunger or increased work of breathing.

- *Chest wall receptors.* Muscle spindles and Golgi apparatus in the muscles of the chest wall function as stretch receptors, monitor 'force generation' and can detect reduced chest wall expansion, thereby contributing to dyspnoea.

Neuroventilatory dissociation

This refers to a situation where there is a mismatch between the information to the central nervous system and afferent muscle activity. For example, in neuromuscular weakness the neural effort is disproportionate to the small amount of muscle movement occurring. Alternatively, in restrictive and obstructive lung disease the neuromuscular effort may be disproportionate to the tidal volume actually achieved. If this happens it has been shown to increase dyspnoea.[23]

Deconditioning

Deconditioning lowers the threshold at which the muscles used in respiration produce lactic acidosis, causing increased respiratory neural output to reduce carbon dioxide levels.

COPD

Many factors contribute to dyspnoea in COPD:

- Hypoxaemia can stimulate peripheral chemoreceptors, increasing ventilatory drive from the brainstem.

- Hypercapnia can directly cause 'air hunger' but also increased central ventilatory drive (to blow off carbon dioxide) and corollary discharge, as discussed above.

- Increased airways resistance and hyperinflation increase the load

---

the respiratory muscles must work against, thereby stimulating muscle receptors.

- Deconditioning via increased lactic acidosis can further contribute to dyspnoea.

Anaemia

It is still unclear what causes dyspnoea in anaemia. It is suspected that, in response to reduced blood oxygen levels, the body 'produces' tachycardia, leading to increased left ventricular end-diastolic pressure. This raised pressure then backs up into the lungs, producing an interstitial oedema that reduces lung compliance and stimulates pulmonary receptors.[27]

Alternatively, it has been suggested that a lack of oxygen produces localised metabolic acidosis and stimulation of 'ergoreceptors' (afferent receptors sensitive to the metabolic effects of muscular work).[28,29]

Heart failure

Heart failure may cause dyspnoea via two mechanisms: interstitial oedema stimulating pulmonary receptors (C-fibres), or hypoxaemia. The first cause (interstitial oedema) is the main mechanism. Interstitial fluid decreases lung compliance (which is picked up by pulmonary C-fibres) and increases the work of breathing.

Asthma

The mechanism of dyspnoea in asthma is thought to be related to an increased *sense of effort and stimulation of irritant airway receptors in the lungs.*[24]

- Bronchoconstriction and airway oedema increase the work of breathing and thus the sensation of effort.

- If hyperinflation occurs, this can change the shape of the diaphragm, affecting stretch of inspiratory muscles, making contraction less efficient and increasing mechanical load. This may lead to increased respiratory motor output and an increased sense of effort.[23]

- Irritation of airway receptors is transmitted by the vagus nerve to the CNS and perceived as chest tightness or constriction.[24]

Neuromuscular disorders

In neuromuscular disorders, central output stimulating respiration is normal; however, muscular strength is often diminished and/or the nerves stimulating the muscles may be weak or damaged. Additional central neural drive is required to activate the weakened muscles[23] and is sensed as increased respiratory effort and dyspnoea.

Pulmonary hypertension

Dyspnoea, particularly on exertion, is very common in primary pulmonary hypertension. The mechanism is dependent on the underlying aetiology.

In chronic pulmonary thrombo-embolism disease (see Figure 1.15), it is thought that pressure receptors or C-fibres in the pulmonary vasculature or right atrium are

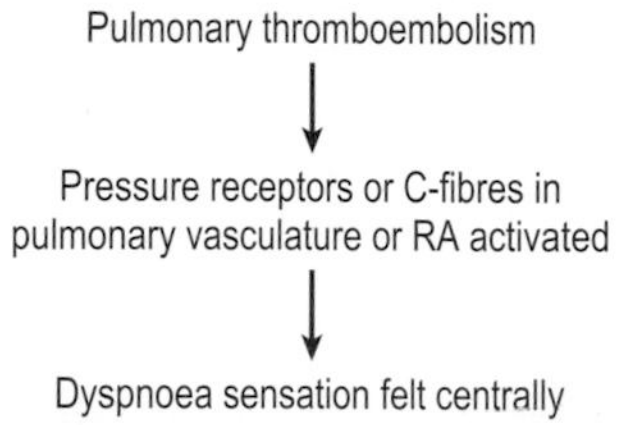

Pulmonary thromboembolism

↓

Pressure receptors or C-fibres in
pulmonary vasculature or RA activated

↓

Dyspnoea sensation felt centrally

FIGURE 1.15
Mechanism of dyspnoea in pulmonary
embolism

activated and interact with central
systems, contributing to dyspnoea.[45]

Primary pulmonary hypertension mechanism/s

Studies of primary pulmonary
hypertension[45,46] have found several
physiological changes that contribute
to dyspnoea. These are depicted in
Figure 1.16:[46]

- relative hypoperfusion of
  ventilated alveoli leading to
  increased V/Q mismatch and
  increased alveolar dead space
- lactic academia occurring at a
  lower-than-normal rate

- hypoxaemia
- inability to increase pulmonary
  blood flow (and therefore
  systemic blood flow) to meet
  exercise oxygen demand.

Sign value

Although a non-specific finding in
isolation, dyspnoea at rest does
require attention. It is often the most
common feature found in patients
with chronic cardiac and lung
conditions.

Recent studies[30] showed the
sensitivity, specificity and positive
predictive value of dyspnoea at rest to
be 92% (95% CI = 90–94%), 19%
(95% CI = 14–24%) and 79% (95%
CI = 77–82%), respectively, in
patients with heart failure. Patients
with dyspnoea at rest were 13% (LR
= 1.13; 95% CI = 1.06–1.20) more
likely to have heart failure than those
without.

Given the low specificity of
dyspnoea and its subjectivity, its value
lies in combining it with other
clinical features.[24]

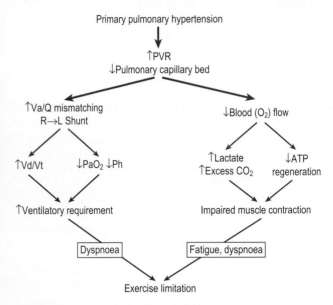

FIGURE 1.16
Pathophysiology of exercise limitation of PPH patients
Longer arrows show pathways leading to dyspnoea and fatigue with exercise. Shorter arrows indicate how each response differs from normal. PVR = pulmonary vascular resistance; Va/Q = alveolar ventilation/perfusion ratio; R = right; L = left; Vd/Vt = dead space volume/tidal volume ratio; PaO_2 = arterial O_2 pressure.

Sun X-G et al. Exercise physiology in patients with primary pulmonary hypertension. Circulation *2001; 104: p. 434, Fig 4.*

Grunting

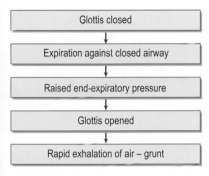

FIGURE 1.17
Mechanism of grunting

Description

A short, explosive, moaning or crying sound heard on expiration, usually in children or neonates.[47]

Condition/s associated with

Any cause of respiratory distress including, but not limited to:

More common

- Paediatric
- Respiratory distress syndrome (hyaline membrane disease) – most common cause
- Meconium aspiration
- Pneumonia
- Congestive heart failure

Less common

- Sepsis
- Heart failure

Mechanism/s

In patients presenting with intrathoracic disease, lower respiratory tract involvement, obstruction or collapse, grunting actually represents an attempt to increase the functional residual capacity.

The patient forcibly expires against a closed glottis and, in doing so, raises end-expiratory pressure. This helps keep narrowed or collapsing airways open, creating a longer time period for the exchange of oxygen and carbon dioxide at the alveoli.[48] The sound of the grunt is caused by the explosive flow of air that occurs when the glottis opens.

Sign value

Grunting is a very valuable sign associated with severe respiratory distress and requires immediate attention.

Haemoptysis

Description

Coughing or spitting up of blood originating from the lungs or bronchial tubes.[49]

Condition/s associated with

There are many potential reasons for haemoptysis. Causes include, but are not limited to:

More common

- Infection – bronchitis, pneumonia, tuberculosis
- Cancer
- Pulmonary embolism
- Foreign body
- Airway trauma
- Idiopathic
- Pulmonary venous hypertension

Less common

- Hereditary haemorrhagic telangiectasia
- Coagulopathy
- Wegener's granulomatosis
- Goodpasture's syndrome

Mechanism/s

The common pathway to haemoptysis is disruption of and damage to vascular systems.

Cancer

Neoplasms produce haemoptysis via invasion of superficial mucosa and erosion into blood vessels. It can also be caused by a highly vascular tumour with fragile vessel walls.[49]

Pulmonary venous hypertension

Any condition that results in pulmonary venous hypertension may cause haemoptysis. For example, left ventricular failure can lead to increasingly high pulmonary venous pressures. These high pressures damage venous walls, causing blood excursion into the lung and eventually haemoptysis.

Infection

Inflammation of lung tissue can disrupt arterial and venous structures. Repetitive cough may damage the pulmonary vasculature, leading to haemoptysis.

Sign value

Although not specific to any one disorder, and bearing in mind that it must be clinically distinguished from haematemesis and other nasal or oral sources of bleeding, haemoptysis always requires investigation.

Hyperventilation

Description

Breathing that occurs in excess of metabolic requirements,[50] usually with an associated tachypnoea.

Condition/s associated with

There are many causes of hyperventilation. They can be broken down into three main categories:

- Psychogenic
  - » Anxiety
  - » Panic attacks

- Organic
  - » Asthma
  - » Pneumonia
  - » Bronchiectasis
  - » COPD
  - » Fibrosing alveolitis
  - » Pulmonary embolus
  - » Pain
  - » CNS disorders
  - » Hepatic disease
- Physiological
  - » Metabolic acidosis
  - » Pregnancy

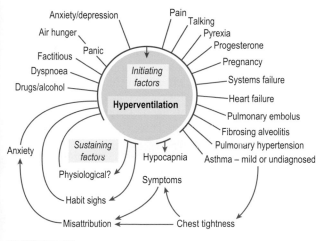

FIGURE 1.18
Factors involved in hyperventilation
Based on Gardner WN, Chest 1996; 109: 516–34.

Mechanism/s

There are many psychological and physical factors that can induce hyperventilation. Figure 1.18 (courtesy of Gardner)[50] demonstrates the different elements at play. A complete understanding of mechanisms for all aetiologies of hyperventilation is not generally necessary; however, there are some key components worth knowing.

Psychogenic

Hyperventilation may induce (as well as be induced by) feelings of anxiety. In patients with anxiety disorders, there is a predisposition to 'over-breathe' based on biological vulnerability, personality and cognitive variables.[51] For example, anxious patients may interpret non-specific chest pain as a heart attack, causing them to attach increased importance to the pain, stimulating the sympathetic nervous system and inducing tachypnoeas and hyperventilation. There is also evidence that these patients may have increased chemoreceptor sensitivity to carbon dioxide and, therefore, are more likely to over-breathe in response to a minor increase in carbon dioxide levels.

In panic disorders, the mechanism is unclear. As for anxiety, hyperventilation may induce a panic attack and vice versa. It is possible that there is a misinterpretation of physiological variables, leading to the brain believing suffocation is taking place, therefore inducing

inappropriate hyperventilation as a response.[52]

Organic causes

Respiratory disease

The most researched example is asthma and, even so, the mechanism is inexact. Suggested contributing mechanism/s include:

- hypoxia stimulating hyperventilation via chemoreceptors
- hyperinflation causing stimulation of pulmonary receptors
- misinterpretation of symptoms – chest pain = heart attack, leading to a sympathetic response, tachypnoeas and hyperventilation (similar to anxiety).

Pulmonary embolism

In pulmonary embolism, the primary mechanism of hyperventilation is thought to be hypoxic drive via chemoreceptors.

CNS disorders

Brainstem injuries may cause altered breathing patterns (see 'Ataxic breathing' and 'Apneustic breathing' in this chapter and 'Cheyne–Stokes breathing' in Chapter 2), most likely due to damage to the ventilatory centres. Hyperventilation has been associated with lesions in the pons, medulla and midbrain.

Hepatic disease

Idiopathic hyperventilation in patients with liver cirrhosis is well described and different from the arterial hypoxia and shortness of breath seen in hepatopulmonary syndrome.

Increased progesterone and oestradiol is well described in cirrhotic patients, owing to impaired breakdown. Progesterone is known to stimulate ventilation receptors in the central nervous system and hyperventilation.[53] Studies have shown a possible relationship between the increased progesterone and ventilation seen in cirrhotic patients, which may represent a possible mechanism for some degree of hyperventilation seen in cirrhotic patients.[54] Progesterone may also increase carbon dioxide sensitivity in cirrhotic patients, making them more prone to hyperventilation.

Physiological causes

Metabolic acidosis

Metabolic acidosis is a well-known cause of tachypnoea as the body attempts to 'blow off' carbon dioxide to reduce acidosis. It is an appropriate response to metabolic requirements and could be thought of in this way as opposed to grouping it with hyperventilation.

Pregnancy

During pregnancy, raised circulating progesterone combines with oestrogen to increase sensitivity to hypoxia, inducing increased ventilation by acting centrally and via the carotid body.[55]

1

Intercostal recession

Description
This refers to the indrawn skin and soft tissue that can be seen in the intercostal spaces on inspiration during times of respiratory distress.

Condition/s associated with
Any form of respiratory distress including, but not limited to:

Common
- Hyaline membrane disease
- Pneumonia
- Bronchiolitis
- Anaphylaxis
- Croup
- Epiglottitis
- Foreign body inhalation

Mechanism/s
In times of increased respiratory effort or respiratory distress, there is increasingly negative intrathoracic pressure, pulling in the skin and soft tissues.

At these times, the accessory muscles are in use and there is a decrease in intrathoracic pressure above that present in normal inspiration. This decreased pressure 'sucks' skin and soft tissue inwards on inspiration, causing intercostal recession.

Sign value
Like accessory muscle usage, it is a non-specific sign of increased work of breathing, but nonetheless very important to notice and useful in monitoring in terms of whether treatment is improving the respiratory status of the patient.

CLINICAL PEARL

Kussmaul's breathing

Description

Also described as 'air hunger', Kussmaul's breathing is typified by deep, rapid inspirations.

Condition/s associated with

Potentially any cause of metabolic acidosis.

More common

- Diabetic ketoacidosis
- Sepsis
- Lactic acidosis

Less common

- Severe haemorrhage
- Uraemia/renal failure
- Renal tubule acidosis (RTA)
- Salicylate poisoning
- Ethylene glycol poisoning
- Biliary/pancreatic fistulas
- Diarrhoea

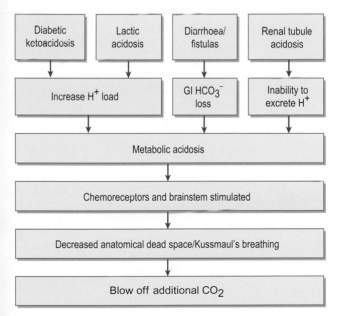

FIGURE 1.19
Kussmaul's respiration mechanism

Mechanism/s

Kussmaul's breathing is an adaptive response to metabolic acidosis. By producing deep, rapid inspirations, anatomical dead space is minimised, allowing for more efficient 'blowing off' of carbon dioxide, thus decreasing acidosis and increasing pH.

Sign value

Although only a few studies have assessed the evidence base for Kussmaul's respiration, it is generally accepted that it is a useful sign. In children, an abnormal respiratory pattern like Kussmaul's respiration has been shown to be a very good sign of 5% or greater dehydration with a likelihood ratio of 2.0.[56]

Orthopnoea

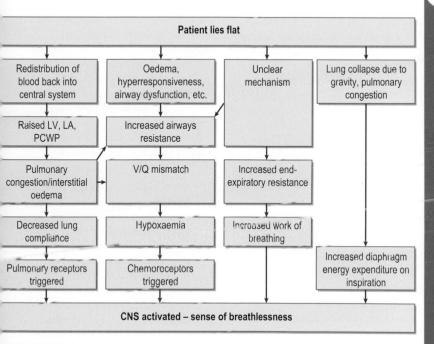

FIGURE 1.20
Mechanism of orthopnoea
LV = left ventricular; LA = left atrial; PCWP = pulmonary capillary wedge pressure.

Description

Dyspnoea that is made worse by lying in a supine position.

Although more often described as a symptom, as sleep studies become more common orthopnoea is increasingly being clinically observed. In either case, it is a useful discovery as the mechanism behind orthopnoea can assist understanding of underlying conditions.

Condition/s associated with

- Congestive heart failure (CHF)
- Bilateral diaphragm paralysis
- COPD
- Asthma

Congestive heart failure mechanism/s

Despite the fact that orthopnoea has been described in medicine for many years, its origin is still not absolutely clear. Figure 1.20 summarises the theories put forward to date.

The current accepted hypothesis for the triggering of orthopnoea is the redistribution of fluid from the splanchnic circulation and lower extremities into the central circulation which occurs while lying flat.[57]

In patients with impaired left ventricular function, the additional blood volume that is returned to the heart cannot be pumped out efficiently. Left ventricular, left atrial and, eventually, pulmonary capillary wedge pressure rises, resulting in pulmonary oedema, increased airways resistance, reduced lung compliance, stimulation of pulmonary receptors and, ultimately, dyspnoea.

Furthermore, replacement of air in the lungs with blood or interstitial fluid can cause a reduction of vital capacity, restrictive physiology and air trapping as a result of small airways closure.[57]

Alterations in the distribution of ventilation and perfusion result in relative V/Q mismatch, with consequent widening of the alveolar–arterial oxygen gradient, hypoxaemia and increased dead space.

Oedema of the bronchial walls can lead to small airways obstruction and produce wheezing ('cardiac asthma').[57]

When lying flat venous return is increased to the heart, increasing end-diastolic volume and pressure. The failing heart is unable to accommodate the increased venous return. End-diastolic pressures rise and are transmitted to the lungs, exacerbating a number of the above factors, and therefore producing orthopnoea.

Recent studies have found other factors that may contribute to orthopnoea in CHF patients:

- *Increased airflow resistance.* Studies have shown that airflow resistance is increased in patients with CHF when lying supine.[58] The reason for this is unclear. It may be due to increased airway hyper-responsiveness and/or airway dysfunction, bronchial mucosal swelling, thickening of the bronchial wall, peribronchial swelling and increased bronchial vein volume,[59] and loss of lung expansion forces due to loss of lung volume.

- *Increased expiratory flow limitation.* There is an increase in expiratory flow limitation in patients with CHF and this is aggravated when they lie flat,[59] making it more difficult for them to expel air from their lungs. Again, the cause of this is not clear. It is possible that when patients lie flat they lose more lung volume (as gravity collapses the lung), further impeding the ability to inspire and expire effectively. Another explanation is that blood redistributing in the lungs affects lung mechanics and increases the expiratory flow limitation.

- *Increased diaphragmatic energy expenditure.*[60] In patients with CHF who are lying flat, there appears to be a rise in diaphragmatic energy expenditure to help deal with the rise in resistive loads to the lung (which the inspiratory muscles must overcome). This increase in the work of the diaphragm also leads to orthopnoea.

Bilateral diaphragm paralysis mechanism/s

Bilateral diaphragm paralysis is a relatively rare cause of orthopnoea, but its presence can lead to prominent, immediate orthopnoea. Pathological states such as amyotrophic lateral sclerosis, trauma, spinal cord disease and multiple sclerosis lead to interruption or destruction of the phrenic nerve or its impulses, which stimulate the diaphragm to contract. When supine, the patient's abdominal contents move towards the head (due to gravity), resulting in decreased residual volume and severe dyspnoea. The diaphragm is unable to contract so cannot push the abdominal contents down.[61–63]

Orthopnoea due to bilateral diaphragm paralysis can be differentiated from that of congestive heart failure by its speed of onset (faster than congestive failure) and the presence of paradoxical abdominal movements.

COPD mechanism/s

Increased inspiratory effort owing to intrinsic PEEP and *increased airways resistance* in the supine position is proposed to contribute to orthopnoea in COPD.[64]

The destruction of lung architecture and premature airway closure on expiration, increased airway resistance and airway collapsibility present in COPD patients result in expiratory flow limitation at rest; that is, expiratory flow is at its maximum during tidal breathing and the only way it can be increased is by breathing at higher lung volumes (i.e. breathing at levels towards total lung capacity).[65]

One of the results of decreased expiratory flow is promotion of dynamic hyperinflation. This is a process where the COPD patient (who is already operating at higher lung volumes than normal), traps more gas as they breathe. This happens due to either increased respiratory rate and therefore decreased time to expire the gas, or increased flow limitation (mentioned above). This generates intrinsic PEEP or increased alveolar pressure at end expiration. As a result of higher end-expiratory pressures, more work is required to take in air on inspiration.

Dynamic flow limitation is exacerbated by lying flat, as is tidal breathing. It thus may contribute to hyperinflation, intrinsic PEEP, inspiratory work[65] and the development of orthopnoea. See Figure 1.21.

Sign value

Orthopnoea is a valuable sign and relatively specific for congestive heart failure. Studies have shown a sensitivity of 42.8% and specificity of 87.51%, with a positive predictive value (PPV) of 14.5% and negative predictive value (NPV) of 96.9%.[66] As in paroxysmal nocturnal dyspnoea (PND), if the sign is absent, it can help exclude heart failure as a cause of breathlessness.

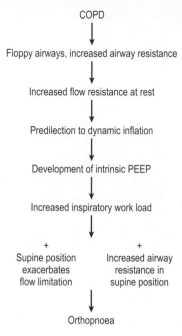

FIGURE 1.21
Mechanism of orthopnoea in COPD

Percussion

The *act* of percussion is obviously not a sign; however, understanding its basis will aid interpretation of particular percussion notes, which *are* signs.

Percussion is traditionally said to produce three distinctive sounds:

1 tympany
2 resonance/hyper-resonance
3 dullness.

Different pathologies underlie the sounds that result from percussion of relevant organs. There are two theoretical mechanisms put forward to explain these sounds – the topographic percussion theory and the cage resonance theory. Anyone other than a respiratory physician would not be expected to know either, but they may assist the diligent percussor to better understand what they are doing and why.

Topographic percussion theory
The central idea in this theory is that only the physical characteristics of *tissues directly underneath* the percussive 'strike' determine the resulting sound. The body wall between the organ and percussor is not acknowledged as contributory, and the sound itself represents structures only to a depth of 4–6 cm underneath the location percussed.[67]

Cage resonance theory
Cage resonance theory states that the percussive note represents the *ease with which the body wall vibrates*. This is affected by the strength of the percussion strike, the state of the body wall and the *underlying organs*. Disease sites *distant* from the percussion strike *can* influence the note heard.[67]

Despite enthusiasm for the topographic percussion theory, the available evidence strongly supports cage resonance as the most likely mechanism.

Percussion: dullness

Description

On percussion of the chest wall and lung fields, a shorter, dull sound of high frequency is heard.

Condition/s associated with

- Pleural effusions
- Pneumonia

Mechanism/s

Pleural fluid dampens the normal resonance of the lung fields, creating the characteristic 'stony' dullness.

Sign value

Only a few variable quality studies exist for dullness of percussion as a sign. One review of three studies[68] found dullness to conventional percussion one of the best signs for predicting the presence of a significant pleural effusion, albeit with a wide confidence interval (positive LR, 8.7; 95% CI, 2.2–33.8). Diacon[69] et al. compared clinical examination to chest ultrasound in locating pleural puncture sites with a resulting sensitivity of 76%, specificity of 60%, positive predictive value of 85% and negative predictive value of 45%. When compared to standard chest radiography, the accuracy with regard to pleural effusion is said to be similar.[70]

Percussion: resonance/ hyper-resonance

Description

Low-pitched hollow sounds traditionally elicited over the lungs. Hyper-resonant sounds are louder and lower pitched than resonant sounds.

Condition/s associated with

- Normal lung fields – resonant
- Pneumothorax – hyper-resonant
- COPD – hyper-resonant

Mechanism/s

In hyper-resonance, over-inflated lungs allow better transmission of the low-frequency sound produced by the percussive tap.

Sign value

Hyper-resonance has been shown to have a PLR of 3.0 to 5.1 in detecting patients with chronic airflow obstruction.[71,72] It has a sensitivity and specificity of 42% and 86% respectively.[72]

In a study of 375 patients, hyper-resonance to percussion was the strongest predictor of COPD, with a sensitivity of only 20.8, but a specificity of 97.8, and likelihood ratio of 9.5.[73] After multivariate logistic regression, where pack-years, shortness of breath, and chest findings were among the explanatory variables, three physical chest findings were independent predictors of COPD, of which hyper-resonance to percussion yielded the highest odds ratio (OR = 6.7).

On a more practical level, hyper-resonance is extremely useful if a post-procedural patient develops shortness of breath or in any acute respiratory distress scenario prior to chest x-ray. Hyper-resonance in these settings requires assessment and management without delay (e.g. pneumothorax).

Platypnoea/orthodeoxia

Description

Platypnoea or 'flat breathing' refers to shortness of breath while sitting or standing that is relieved by lying supine. It is the opposite of orthopnoea. Orthodeoxia refers to arterial desaturation noted when sitting up as opposed to lying down. These are not common signs but are quite striking when present.

Condition/s associated with

- Cardiac (intracardiac shunt)
  » Atrial septal defect (ASD)
  » Patent foramen ovale (PFO)
  » Pneumonectomy

  Usually associated with pulmonary hypertension or raised right atrial (RA) pressure (e.g. constrictive pericarditis, cardiac tamponade).

- Pulmonary (intrapulmonary right-to-left shunts)
  » Hepatopulmonary syndrome
  » Pulmonary diseases
  » COPD
  » Pulmonary embolism

- Upper airway tumour
  » Acute respiratory distress syndrome

- Miscellaneous causes
  » Autonomic neuropathy
  » Acute respiratory distress syndrome (ARDS)

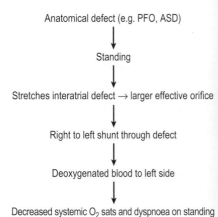

Anatomical defect (e.g. PFO, ASD)

↓

Standing

↓

Stretches interatrial defect → larger effective orifice

↓

Right to left shunt through defect

↓

Deoxygenated blood to left side

↓

Decreased systemic O_2 sats and dyspnoea on standing

FIGURE 1.22
Simplified mechanism of platypnoea/orthodeoxia

Cheng TO, Platypnea-orthodeoxia syndrome: etiology, differential diagnosis and management. Catheterization and Cardiovascular Interventions; *1999: 47: 64–66.*

General mechanism/s

In general, *shunting of blood from the venous to the arterial system* can result in platypnoea/orthodeoxia. There are multiple ways in which this shunting may transpire and they are complex.[74] For simplicity they may be divided into three categories: intracardiac shunts, pulmonary arteriovenous shunts or ventilation/perfusion mismatching.[75]

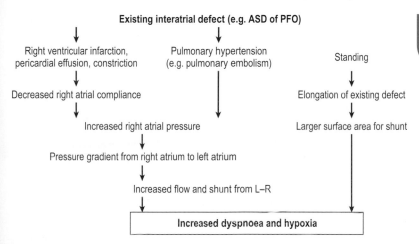

FIGURE 1.23
Mechanism of platypnoea/orthodeoxia

Cheng TO, Platypnea-orthodeoxia syndrome: etiology, differential diagnosis and management.
Catheterization and Cardiovascular Interventions; *1999: 47: 64–66.*

Intracardiac shunts (e.g. patent foramen ovale)

Under normal circumstances, the presence of a communication between the left and right sides of the heart would lead to left to right shunting, given that systemic pressures are higher than right-sided and pulmonary pressures. Bearing this in mind, it is proposed that a *second* functional and/or positional abnormality in/directly contributes to 'pushing' blood across the defect in a *right to left* shunt – resulting in platypnoea/orthodeoxia.[76]

Platypnoea may occur in patients with an isolated PFO or in patients with a PFO *and* secondary raised right atrial pressure. This is demonstrated in Figure 1.23. Some patients who demonstrate platypnoea in the presence of a PFO may undergo a postural redirection of inferior vena cava (IVC) blood flow towards the atrial septum and left atrium.[74] Standing upright may stretch the interatrial communication (PFO) and allow for more streaming of venous blood from the IVC through the defect.

Changes in right atrial compliance and pressure may also facilitate increased right to left shunting and the development of platypnoea/orthodeoxia. For example, right ventricular infarction, pulmonary embolism, constrictive pericarditis or pericardial effusion can decrease right atrial compliance and increase pressure, which will contribute to further propulsion of blood across the existing defect.

Pneumonectomy

Pneumonectomy may cause increased right-sided pressures of the heart. The rise is due to the smaller pulmonary vascular bed present with a single lung. In time, the right ventricle may become less compliant than the left, elevating RV and RA pressures and producing a pressure gradient across the atrial septal defect (ASD) or PFO, resulting in a right-to-left shunt and platypnoea.

Pulmonary arteriovenous shunts

Pulmonary arteriovenous malformations have been associated with platypnoea/orthodeoxia and are usually located in the lung bases. It is thought that when the patient sits or stands upright, increased blood flow through the basal malformations or shunts occurs due to gravity, leading to increased deoxygenated blood going to the left side of the heart, causing dyspnoea and hypoxaemia.

Hepatic

Platypnoea in liver disease is predominantly due to intrapulmonary shunting of deoxygenated blood and V/Q mismatch. The mechanism for this is multifaceted as hepatopulmonary syndrome has been shown to cause numerous pulmonary system changes which can result in altered oxygenation:[74]

- Diffuse intrapulmonary shunts are formed, mainly by pre-capillary and capillary vascular dilatations (some arteriovenous anastamoses are seen as well).[77]

- Impaired hypoxic vasoconstriction leads to deoxygenated blood

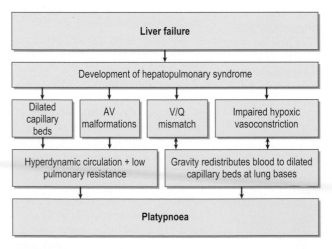

FIGURE 1.24
Mechanism of platypnoea in hepatopulmonary syndrome

passing through areas of poor gas exchange rather than being redistributed to areas of better ventilation.

- Development or worsening of V/Q mismatch.
- Pleural effusions and diaphragmatic dysfunction.

In addition to these factors, it is thought that while sitting up allows gravity to redistribute blood to the lung bases, where there are dilated pre-capillary beds, this also means that less oxygenation of blood occurs, producing hypoxaemia and dyspnoea.

It has also been shown that patients with hepatopulmonary syndrome have a hyperdynamic circulation and low pulmonary resistance, meaning there is less time for deoxygenated blood to become oxygenated in the lungs.

Pulmonary ventilation/ perfusion (V/Q) mismatching

Like the cardiac causes, pulmonary origins of platypnoea involve *deoxygenated blood being shunted to the arterial system.*

It is suggested that lung disease causes changes in lung mechanics, raised alveolar pressures, decreased pulmonary artery pressures leading to pulmonary artery compression and increased respiratory dead space[78] – all of which worsen V/Q mismatch and/or intrapulmonary shunts, resulting in platypnoea. When the patient is standing upright, right ventricular preload is reduced, resulting in lower output to the pulmonary arteries to the extent that alveolar pressure exceeds arterial and venous pressures. The upshot of this is that minimal blood flow is oxygenated and ventilated. Adding to this, standing and gravity cause more blood to flow to the basal segments of the lung, worsening the V/Q mismatch and causing increased dyspnoea.[75]

Sign value

Platypnoea is a rare but valuable sign; if seen it almost certainly indicates a pathology causing a shunt of blood from the venous to the arterial system.

Pursed-lip breathing (PLB)

Description

A breathing practice, often taught, which includes a long, slow expiration against pursed lips.

Condition/s associated with

- COPD

Mechanism/s

To understand the reason for pursed-lip breathing the pathophysiology behind chronic obstructive pulmonary disease must be appreciated. Inflammation of the airways ultimately leads to destruction of lung parenchyma and emphysema. The resultant reduction in elastic recoil, along with fibrosis and muscle hypertrophy, causes increased airways resistance and premature airway closing on expiration or *expiratory airflow limitation*. This results in air trapping at end expiration and, with time, hyperinflation. When coupled with periods of increased respiratory rate (during which the relative expiratory phase of respiration is short), dynamic hyperinflation occurs.

Pursing the lips allows the patient to *breathe against resistance*, thus maintaining a slow exhalation pressure within the lungs. This helps keep bronchioles and small airways open for much-needed oxygen exchange.[79,80] As such, it allows deeper breathing and improved V/Q matching.

PLB has been shown to have other physiological benefits:

- reduction in breathing frequency, a longer relative expiratory time and a reduction in intrinsic PEEP (i.e. gas trapping), and therefore less dynamic hyperinflation
- increased tidal volume
- increased expiratory airway pressure and therefore a reduction in expiratory airways collapse, expiratory flow limitation and airways resistance.[81]

Sign value

Pursed-lip breathing has become a therapeutic modality in patients with COPD to help alleviate dyspnoea. It has been shown to reduce respiratory rate and increase efficacy of ventilation, tidal volume and oxygen saturation.[82,83]

Sputum

Description

Matter/mucus ejected from the lungs, bronchi and trachea through the mouth.

Condition/s associated with

- COPD
- Pneumonia
- Tuberculosis (TB)
- Bronchiectasis
- Malignancy
- Cystic fibrosis
- Asthma

Mechanism/s

Mucus is produced by glands within the tracheobronchial tree. Irritants such as cigarette smoke or inflammation increase mucus production. Inflammation and irritation from a variety of causes can stimulate the cough reflex (see entry in this chapter) to bring up sputum.

Sign value

A very non-specific sign if produced in isolation from other signs, symptoms or history. However, a recent change in colour or quantity of sputum is worth investigating. Studies have shown:

- Sputum culture samples are of limited value in COPD unless the patient is not responding to antibiotics.[84]

- In patients with COPD, the presence of green (purulent) sputum was 94.4% sensitive and 77.0% specific for the yield of a high bacterial load, allowing timely identification of those who require antibiotics.[85]

- For patients producing white, cream or clear coloured sputum, bacterial count was low and further testing was not warranted.[86]

- In the Australian COPDX guidelines, an increased volume and/or change of colour of sputum is used as a marker for an infective exacerbation of COPD.

- There is debate over the value of sputum and sputum Gram stain and cultures in community-acquired pneumonia.[87] One recent study[88] found sputum Gram stain to be a dependable test for early diagnosis of bacterial community-acquired pneumonia. This can assist with rational and appropriate initial antimicrobial therapy. However, there is a financial cost to the test and given that most community-acquired pneumonias are caused by streptococcus pneumonia, it may be argued that it is better to treat empirically and only test high-risk or difficult-to-treat cases.

- In tuberculosis endemic areas, sputum collection is a key tool in diagnosis and management. The diagnostic value of 'rust-coloured' sputum in TB is not clear. Microscopic examination of sputum is required.

Stridor

Description

Stridor (from the Latin *stridere*, 'to creak') is a loud, intense, monophasic sound with constant pitch. It is best heard over the extrathoracic airways and is most commonly inspiratory, but may be expiratory or biphasic in timing if a lesion below the level of the larynx is present.

Condition/s associated with

Any form of upper airway obstruction.

More common

- Foreign body
- Croup
- Peritonsillar abscess
- Aspiration

Less common

- Laryngomalacia – chronic, low-pitched stridor, most common form of inspiratory stridor in neonates
- Subglottic stenosis – chronic, common form of biphasic stridor
- Vocal cord dysfunction – chronic, common form of biphasic stridor
- Laryngeal haemangiomas
- Tracheomalacia and bronchiomalacia – expiratory stridor
- Epiglottitis

TABLE 1.3
Type of stridor and location of obstruction

Stridor type	Obstruction location
Inspiratory	Laryngeal/supraglottic lesion
Expiratory	Tracheobronchial lesion – below thoracic inlet
Biphasic	Subglottic/glottic to tracheal ring

Mechanism/s

Any obstruction in the extrathoracic airways (supraglottis, glottis, subglottis and/or trachea) causes *narrowing and flow turbulence*. In addition, as with stertor, narrowing causes an increase in flow velocity and a pressure drop across the narrowing, causing further narrowing or temporary closure of the airway, contributing to the production of the sound (see Table 1.3).

Characteristics of stridor

The volume, pitch and phase of stridor can be helpful if attempting to localise the obstruction:[89]

- *Volume:* stridor is believed to represent a significant narrowing of the airway,[89] but a sudden drop in volume may indicate impending airway collapse.[90]

- *Pitch:*
  - » High-pitched stridor is usually caused by obstruction at the level of the glottis.[91]
  - » Lower-pitched stridor is often caused by higher lesions in the nose, nasopharynx and supraglottic larynx.[92]
  - » Intermediate pitch usually signifies obstruction at the subglottis or below.[92]
- *Phase:*
  - » Inspiratory – the obstruction is usually above the glottis.[93]
  - » Biphasic – fixed obstruction at the glottis or subglottis down to tracheal ring.[89]
  - » Expiratory – suggests collapse of the lower airways below the thoracic inlet.[89]

Sign value

Stridor is a valuable sign that can quickly identify upper airways obstruction. Once heard it is never forgotten. It must be investigated and managed quickly.

Tachypnoea

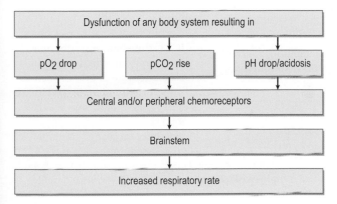

FIGURE 1.25
Simplified mechanism of tachypnoea

Description

A respiratory rate measured above 20 breaths per minute.

Condition/s associated with

Tachypnoea may be produced by many different system pathologies including:

- Cardiac
- Respiratory
- CNS
- Infectious
- Psychogenic
- Pain

Mechanism/s

Any state causing a derangement in oxygen (hypoxia), pCO_2 (hypercapnia) or acid/base status (acidosis) will stimulate respiratory drive and increase respiratory rate.

Tachypnoea occurs *in most situations as a compensatory response to either a drop in pO_2 (hypoxaemia) or a rise in pCO_2 (hypercapnia)*. Central chemoreceptors in the medulla and peripheral chemoreceptors in the aortic arch and carotid body measure a combination of these variables and send messages to the central ventilatory systems to increase respiratory rate and tidal volume to compensate for any fluctuations.[94]

Sign value

Tachypnoea is a very valuable vital sign and is unfortunately often neglected when routine observations are performed. Studies reviewing tachypnoea have shown:

- Predicting cardiopulmonary arrest – sensitivity of 0.54, specificity of 0.83, odds ratio of 5.56.[95]

- In unstable patients, the change in respiratory rate is better at predicting an at-risk patient than heart rate or blood pressure.[96]

- Unwell patients with a higher respiratory rate had a higher risk of death.[97]

- Over half of all patients suffering a serious adverse event on general hospital wards had a respiratory rate greater than 24 breaths/minute.[98]

- In predicting negative outcomes (ICU admission or death) in community-acquired pneumonia, respiratory rate of greater than 27 had sensitivity of 70%, specificity of 67%, PPV of 27% and NPV of 93%.[94]

New onset or change in rate of tachypnoea requires quick and thorough investigation. It may herald ominous decompensation.

Tracheal tug

Description

Downward displacement of the thyroid cartilage during inspiration.

Condition/s associated with

Most common

- Respiratory distress/COPD (Campbell's sign)

Less common

- Arch of aorta aneurysm (Oliver's sign)

Mechanism/s

Tracheal tug – Campbell's sign

Patients in respiratory distress have increased work of breathing and the *movements of the chest wall, muscles and diaphragm* are transmitted along the trachea, pulling it rhythmically downwards.

An alternative cause of tracheal tug occurs in patients who have *intercostal weakness but preserved diaphragmatic strength*. This can be caused by muscle relaxants and deep sedation from anaesthetic agents and is due to the unopposed action of the crura pulling on the diaphragm, which also pulls the pericardium and lung structures during inspiration.

Tracheal tug – Oliver's sign

Tracheal tug in this situation refers to downward displacement of the cricoid cartilage in time with ventricular contraction, in the presence of an aortic arch aneurysm. With the patient's chin lifted, the clinician can grasp the cricoid cartilage and push it upwards. This movement brings the aortic arch and the aortic aneurysm (if present) closer to the left main bronchus (which it overrides). The pulsation of the aorta and the aneurysm is then transmitted up the bronchus to the trachea, creating Oliver's sign.

Sign value

There is limited evidence as to value; however, tracheal tug is generally accepted as a sign of increased work of breathing.

Oliver's sign is much rarer than the tracheal tug seen with COPD and/or respiratory distress.

Trepopnoea

Description

Dyspnoea which is worse when the patient is lying on one side (in lateral decubitus position), which is relieved by lying on the opposite side.

Condition/s associated with

- Unilateral lung disease
- Congestive heart failure – dilated cardiomyopathy
- Lung tumour

Mechanism/s

Unilateral lung disease

When the patient lies on the side of the 'good' lung, gravity increases blood flow to the lower lung and improves oxygenation.

Congestive heart failure

These patients prefer to lie on their right side. The cause of this preference is as yet unclear.

Recent studies[99] suggest that lying on the right side enhances *venous return and sympathetic activity*. It is also thought that the right lateral position allows changes to the *hydrostatic forces* on the right and left ventricles, which can reduce lung congestion.

Other potential contributing factors include:[100]

- positional improvements in lung mechanics – the enlarged heart is not causing atelectasis by pushing on the lung
- less airway compression
- in patients with decreased compliance of the left ventricle, its compression has a greater impact on filling pressures. This occurs when lying in the left lateral position.

Lung tumour

Gravity causes tumours to compress the lungs and/or vasculature, depending on location. Therefore, a tumour of sufficient size in a significant site can cause a transient V/Q mismatch, hypoxia/hypercarbia and breathlessness.

Sign value

There is limited evidence on the sensitivity and specificity values; however, trepopnoea is pathological and requires investigation. A recent small study has suggested that trepopnoea in heart failure may be more common than initially thought and is present in up to 51% of patients.

Vocal fremitus/tactile fremitus

Description

The vibration felt when placing the hands on the back of a patient and asking them to speak (usually the phrase 'ninety-nine'). The vibration is decreased in bigger areas of air, fat, fluid or tumour, whereas it is increased in areas of consolidation. Symmetrical fremitus may be physiological, whereas asymmetrical fremitus should always be considered abnormal.

Condition/s associated with

- Pneumonia – increased vocal fremitus
- Pneumothorax – decreased fremitus
- Pleural effusion – decreased fremitus
- COPD – decreased fremitus
- Tumour

Mechanism/s

As discussed in 'Vocal resonance' in this chapter, variation in vocal fremitus can be explained by the manner in which various *voice frequencies are transmitted through tissue or fluid*.

In pneumonia, consolidation *augments lower frequencies* (such as the human voice) and thus is more likely to be felt as a stronger vibration. Large pleural effusions decrease the *transmission of low frequencies* and thus diminish vocal fremitus.

Sign value

See box under 'Vocal resonance'.

Vocal resonance

Description

Vocal resonance refers to the character of the patient's voice heard with the stethoscope over the posterior lung fields. Normally a patient's voice is muffled and difficult to understand in this situation but in consolidated areas it will be heard clearly.

Classically, the changes in vocal resonance seen with disease are:

- bronchophony – voice is louder than normal
- pectoriloquy – whispered words are clearly heard, also called 'whispering pectoriloquy'
- aegophony – the voice has a nasal, bleating quality (like a goat); implies high resonance.

Condition/s associated with

Changes in vocal resonance are classically associated with:

Inflammation, consolidation and pus

↓

Transmission of low and high frequencies

↓

Increased vocal resonance

FIGURE 1.26
Mechanism of increased vocal resonance

- Consolidation: tumour, pneumonia
- Pleural effusion

Mechanism/s

The differences in vocal resonance are determined by the *transmission frequency (Hz)* and the physical properties of normal lungs, fluid and consolidation. These elements are common to the mechanism/s of '*breath sounds*'.

Normal lung tissue filters out lower-frequency sounds and transmits high-frequency sounds.[8] Human

---

CLINICAL PEARL

Vocal fremitus versus vocal resonance

Vocal fremitus and resonance are always taught but probably under-utilised as clinical signs. One study[8] looking at pleural effusions showed the following diagnostic utility:

- *Reduced vocal fremitus*: sensitivity 82%, specificity 86%, PPV 0.59, NPV 0.95, PLR 5.67, NLR 0.21
- *Reduced vocal resonance*: sensitivity 76%, specificity 88%, PPV 0.62, NPV 0.94, PLR 6.49, NLR 0.27.

voices are *generally lower in frequency* and, therefore, are not well transmitted.

Consolidated lungs transmit *low and higher frequencies effectively* and so a patient's voice is heard clearly and easily over a consolidated area.

Large effusions (due to the physical properties of fluid) *reduce the transmission of lower frequencies*[9,101,102] and therefore voices are muffled or less audible.

Sign value

In patients with cough and fever, aegophony has very good specificity for detecting pneumonia — sensitivity of 4–16%, specificity of 96–99%.[9]

1

Wheeze

Description

Continual high-pitched 'musical' sounds heard at the end of inspiration or at the start of expiration.

Condition/s associated with

- Asthma
- Respiratory tract infections
- COPD
- Foreign body aspiration: bronchial foreign bodies in children may present with a 'triad' of unilateral wheeze + cough + decreased breath sounds.

Mechanism/s

Airway narrowing allows airflow-induced oscillation of airway walls, producing acoustic waves.[103] As the airway lumen becomes smaller, the airflow velocity increases, resulting in vibration of the airway wall and the tonal quality.

Sign value

A wheeze on normal quiet expiration or inspiration is most likely pathological. The longer and more high pitched the wheeze, the more severe the obstruction is.[104] Changes of extent and pitch[105] should be monitored when assessing response to treatment in chronic obstructive pulmonary disease. Wheeze monitoring has also been used to good effect in assessing asthma severity and response to treatment.[106]

Remember that having a wheeze implies that the patient has enough air movement to produce one. Beware the wheezing patient who suddenly becomes silent, as this may mean air movement is so *low* that a wheeze cannot be produced. If this happens, respiratory arrest may be imminent.

CLINICAL PEARL

Monophonic versus polyphonic wheeze

Monophonic wheeze

A wheeze with a single note that starts and ends at different points in time. The classic example is caused by a tumour in the bronchi. The pitch and timing is fixed as the tumour itself is static.

A child with a fixed foreign body may have a monophonic wheeze.

Polyphonic wheeze

A wheeze with several different tones starting and finishing at the same time. It is heard when a fixed compression occurs in multiple bronchi at the same time. Can be present in COPD and in healthy people at end expiration. It is caused by second- or third-order bronchi closing at the same time at end expiration, as the pressures within the airway keeping them patent are reduced.

References

1. O'Neill S, McCarthy DS. Postural relief of dyspnoea in severe chronic airflow limitation: relationship to respiratory muscle strength. *Thorax* 1983;**38**:595–600.

2. Mattos WL, et al. Accuracy of clinical examination findings in the diagnosis of COPD, but the interrelator reliability was poor. *J Bras Pneumol* 2009;**35**(5):404–8.

3. Perkin RM, Resnik DB. The agony of agonal respirations: is the last gasp necessary? *J Med Ethics* 2002;**28**:164–9.

4. Perkins GD, Walker G, Christensen K, Hulme J, Monsieurs KG. Teaching recognition of agonal breathing improves accuracy of diagnosing cardiac arrest. *Resuscitation* 2006;**70**:432–7.

5. Roppolo LP, Westfall A, Pepe PE, et al. Dispatcher assessments for agonal breathing improve detection of cardiac arrest. *Resuscitation* 2009;**80**(7):769–72.

6. Eckert DJ, Jordan AS, Merchia P, Malhotra A. Central sleep apnoea: pathophysiology and treatment. *Chest* 2007;**131**:595–607.

7. Douglas BT, Phillipson EA. Chapter 74: Sleep disorders. In: Mason RJ, Murray JF, Broaddus VC, Nadal JA, editors. *Murray and Nadal's Respiratory Medicine*. 4th ed. 2010. Available: http://www.mdconsult.com.ezproxy1.library.usyd.edu.au/das/book/body/185300500-5/957919650/1288/689.html#4-u1.0-B0-7216-0327-0..50077-X-cesec7_4145 [28 Feb 2011].

8. Kalantri S, Joshi R, Lokhande T, et al. Accuracy and reliability of physical signs in the diagnosis of pleural effusion. *Respir Med* 2007;**101**:431–8.

9. McGee S. *Evidence Based Physical Diagnosis*. 2nd ed. St Louis: Saunders; 2007.

10. Silbernagl S, Lang F. *Color Atlas of Pathophysiology*. New York: Thieme; 2010. p. 82.

11. Gnitecki J, Moussavi Z. Separating heart sounds from lung sounds. *IEEE Eng Med Biol Mag* 2007;**26**(1):20–9.

12. Loudon R, Murphy RLH. State of the art: lung sounds. *Am Rev Respir Dis* 1984;**130**:663–73.

13. Stahlheber C, et al. Breath sound assessment. Available: http://emedicine.medscape.com/article/1894146-overview#showall [17 Sept 2014].

14. Bohadana A, Izbicki G, Kraman S. Fundamentals of lung auscultation. *NEJM* 2014;**370**(21):744–51.

15. Ceresa CC, Johnston I. Auscultation in the diagnosis of the respiratory disease in the 21st century. *Postgrad Med J* 2008;**84**:393–4.

16. Mangione S. *Physical Diagnosis Secrets*. 2nd ed. St Louis: Elsevier; 2007.

17. Schreur HJ, Sterk PJ, Vanderschoot J, et al. Lung sound intensity in patients with emphysema and in normal subjects at standardised airflows. *Thorax* 1992;**47**:674–9.

18. Gurugn A, et al. Computerized lung sound analysis as diagnostic aid for the detection of abnormal lung sounds: A systematic review and meta-analysis. *Respir Med* 2011;**105**(9):1396–403.

19. Pardee NE, Martin CJ, Morgan EH. A test of the practical value of estimating breath sound intensity. Breath sounds are related to measured ventilatory function. *Chest* 1976;**70**(3):341–4.

20. Gilbert R, Ashutosh K, Auchincloss JH, et al. Prospective study of controlled oxygen therapy: poor prognosis of patients with asynchronous breathing. *Chest* 1977;**71**:456–62.

21. Badgett RG, Tanaka DJ, Hunt DK, et al. Can moderate chronic obstructive pulmonary disease be diagnosed by historical and physical findings alone? *Am J Med* 1993;**94**:188–96.

22. Al Jarad N, Strickland B, Bothamley G, et al. Diagnosis of asbestosis by a time expanded wave form analysis, auscultation and high resolution computed tomography: a comparative study. *Thorax* 1993;**48**:347–53.

23. Scano G, Ambrosino N. Pathophysiology of dyspnoea. *Lung* 2002;**180**:131–48.

24. Manning HL, Schwartzstein RM. Pathophsyiology of dyspnoea. *N Engl J Med* 1995;**133**(23):1547–53.

25. Chanon T, Mullholland MB, Leitner J, Altose MD, Cherniack NS. Sensation of dyspnoea during hypercapnia, exercise and voluntary hyperventilation. *J Appl Physiol* 1990;**68**:2100–6.

26. O'Donnell DE, Sannii R, Anthonisen NR, Younes M. Expiratory resistance loading in patients with severe chronic airflow limitation: an evaluation of ventilatory mechanics and compensatory responses. *Am Rev Resp Dis* 1987;**138**:1185–91.

27. Schwartzstein R, Stoller JK, Hollingsworth H. Physiology of dyspnoea. *Uptodate* November 2009;version 19.1.

28. Clark AL, Peipoli M, Coats AJ. Skeletal muscle and the control of ventilation on exercise: evidence of metabolic receptors. *Eur J Clin Invest* 1996;**25**:299.

29. Clark A, Volterrani M, Swan JW, et al. Leg blood flow, metabolism and exercise in chronic stable heart failure. *Int J Cardiol* 1996;**55**:127.

30. Ahmed A, Allman RM, Aronow WS, DeLong JF. Diagnosis of heart failure in older adults: predictive value of dyspnoea at rest. *Arch Gerontol Geriatr* 2004;**38**(3):297–307.

31. Nakaoka T, Uemura S, Yano T, Nakagawa Y, Tanimoto T, Suehiro S. Does overgrowth of costal cartilage cause pectus excavatum? A study on the lengths of ribs and costal cartilage in asymmetric patients. *J Paediatr Surg* 2009;**44**(7):1333–6.

32. Shamberger RC. Congenital chest wall deformities. *Curr Probl Surg* 1996;**33**(6):469–542.

33. Vyshedskiy A, Alhashem RM, Paciej R, et al. Mechanism of inspiratory and expiratory crackles. *Chest* 2009;**135**(1):156–64.

34. Dalmasso F, et al. A computer system for timing and acoustical analysis of crackles: a study in cryptogenic fibrosing alveolitis. *Bull Eur Physiopathol Respir* 1984;**20**:139–3.

35. Piirila P, Sovijarvi ARA. Crackles: recording, analysis and clinical significance. *Eur Respir J* 1995;**8**:2139–48.

36. Nath AR, Capel LH. Inspiratory crackles – early and late. *Thorax* 1974;**29**:223.

37. Piirila P. *Acoustic properties of cough and crackling lung sounds in patients with pulmonary diseases. Doctoral thesis.* Helsinki: Helsinki University; 1992 ISBN 951-801-900-2.

38. Cottin V, Cordier J-F. Velcro crackles: The key for early diagnosis of idiopathic pulmonary fibrosis? *Eur Respir J* 2012;**40**(3):519–21.

39. McGee S. *Evidence Based Physical Diagnosis*. 3rd ed. St Louis: Elsevier; 2012.

40. Murphy RL Jr, et al. Crackles in the early diagnosis of asbestosis. *Am Rev Respir Dis* 1984;**129**:375–9.

41. Marques A. Are crackles an appropriate outcome measure for airway clearance techniques. *Respir Care* 2012;**57**(9):1468–75.

42. Ponte D, et al. Characterisation of crackles from patients with fibrosis, heart failure and pneumonia. *Med Eng Phys* 2013;**35**:448–56.

43. Flietstra B, et al. Automated analysis of crackles in patients with interstitial pulmonary fibrosis. *Pulm Med* 2011;**2011** doi: 10.1155/2011/590506.

44. Marques A, et al. Computerised adventitious respiratory sounds as outcome measures for respiratory therapy: a systematic review. *Respir Care* 2014;**59**(5):765–76.

45. Sajkov D, Latimer K, Petrovsky N. Dyspnea in pulmonary arterial hypertension, pulmonary hypertension. In: Sulica R, Preston I, editors. *Bench Research to Clinical Challenges, InTech*. 2011. pp. 191–208. Available: http://www.intechopen.com/articles/show/title/dyspnea-in-pulmonary-arterial-hypertension.

46. Sun X-G, et al. Exercise physiology in patients with primary pulmonary hypertension. *Circulation* 2001;**104**:429–35.

47. Mathers LH, Frankel LR. Stabilization of the critically ill child. In: Behrman RE, Kliegman RM, Jenson HB, editors. *Nelson Textbook of Pediatrics*. 17th ed. Philadelphia: WB Saunders; 2003. pp. 279–96.

48. Ely E. Grunting respirations: sure distress. *Nursing* 1989;**19**(3):72–3.

49. Bidwell JL, Pachner RW. Haemoptysis: diagnosis and management. *Am Fam Physician* 2005;**77**(7):1253–60.

50. Gardner WN. The pathophysiology of hyperventilation disorders. *Chest* 1996;**109**:516–34.

51. Bass C, Kartsounis L, Lelliott P. Hyperventilation and its relationship to anxiety and panic. *Integr Psych* 1987;**5**:274–91.

52. Klein DF. False suffocation alarms, spontaneous panics and related conditions. *Arch Gen Psychiatry* 1993;**50**:306–17.

53. Lustik LJ. The hyperventilation of cirrhosis: progesterone and estradiol effects. *Hepatology* 1997;**25**(1):55–8.

54. Passino C, et al. Abnormal hyperventilation in patients with hepatic cirrhosis: role of enhanced chemosensitivity to carbon dioxide. *Int J Cardiol* 2012;**54**(1):22–6.

55. Hannhart B, Pickett CK, Moore LG. Effects of estrogen and progesterone on carotid body neural output responsiveness to hypoxia. *J Appl Physiol* 1990;**68**:1909–16.

56. Steiner MJ, DeWalt DA, Byerley JS. Is this child dehydrated? *JAMA* 2004;**291**:2746–54.

57. Kusumoto FM. Chapter 10: Cardiovascular disorders: heart disease. In: McPhee SJ, Hammer GD, editors. *Pathophysiology of Disease: An Introduction to Clinical Medicine*. 6th ed. 2010. Available: http://www.accesspharmacy.com/content.aspx?aID=5367630 [13 Mar 2011].

58. Yap JC, Moore DM, Cleland JG, et al. Effect of supine posture on respiratory mechanics in chronic left ventricular failure. *Am J Respir Crit Care Med* 2000; **162**(4 Pt 1):1285–91.

59. Duguet A, Tantucci C, Lozinguez O, et al. Expiratory flow limitation as a determinant of orthopnea in acute left heart failure. *J Am Coll Cardiol* 2000;**35**:690–700.

60. Nava S, Larvovere M, Fanfulla F, et al. Orthopnea and inspiratory effort in chronic heart failure patients. *Respir Med* 2003;**97**(6):647–53.

61. Yelgec NS, et al. Severe orthopnea is not always due to heart failure: a case of bilateral diaphragm paralysis. *J Emerg Med* 2013;**45**(6):922–3.

62. Kumar N, Folger WN, Bolton CF. Dyspnea as the predominant manifestation of bilateral phrenic neuropathy. *Mayo Clin Proc* 2004;**79**:1563–5.

63. Celli BR. Respiratory management of diaphragm paralysis. *Semin Respir Crit Care Med* 2002;**23**:275–81.

64. Loubna E, et al. Orthopnea and tidal expiratory flow limitation in patients with stable COPD. *Chest* 2001;**119**(1):99–104.

65. Tantucci C. Expiratory flow limitation definition, mechanisms, methods, and significance. *Pulm Med* 2013;**2013**.

66. Ekundayo OJ, Howard VJ, Safford MM, et al. Value of orthopnea, paroxysmal nocturnal dyspnoea, and medications in prospective population studies of incident heart failure. *Am J Cardiol* 2009;**104**(2):259–64.

67. McGee SR. Percussion and physical diagnosis: separating myth from science. *Dis Mon* 1995;**41**(10):641–92.

68. Wong C, et al. Does this patient have a pleural effusion? *JAMA* 2009;**301**(3):309–17.

69. Diacon AH, Brutsche MH, Soler M. Accuracy of pleural puncture sites: a prospective comparison of clinical examination with ultrasound. *Chest* 2003;**123**:436–41.

70. Diaz-Guzman E, Budev MM. Accuracy of physical examination in evaluating pleural effusion. *Cleve Clin J Med* 2008;**75**(4):297–303.

71. Badgett RG, Tanaka DJ, Hunt DK, et al. Can moderate chronic obstructive pulmonary disease be diagnosed by historical and physical findings alone? *Am J Med* 1993;**94**:188–96.

72. Badgett RG, et al. The clinical evaluation for diagnosing obstructive airways disease in high risk patients. *Chest* 1994;**106**:1427–31.

73. Oshaug K, Halvorsen PA, Melbye H. Should chest examination be reinstated in the early diagnosis of chronic obstructive pulmonary disease? *Int J Chron Obstruct Pulmon Dis* 2013;**8**:369–77.

74. Natalie AA, Nichols L, Bump GM. Platypnea-orthodeoxia, an uncommon presentation of patent foramen ovale. *Am J Med Sci* 2010;**339**(1):78–80.

75. Rodigues P, et al. Platypnea-orthodexia syndrome in review: defining a new disease? *Cardiology* 2012;**123**:15–23.

76. Cheng TO. Platypnea-orthodeoxia syndrome: etiology, differential diagnosis and management. *Catheter Cardiovasc Interv* 1999;**47**:64–6.

77. Rodriguez-Roisin R, Krowka MJ. Hepatopulmonary syndrome – a liver induced lung vascular disorder. *N Engl J Med* 2008;**358**(22):2378–87.

78. Hussain SF, Mekan SF. Platypnea-orthodeoxia: report of two cases and review of the literature. *South Med J* 2004;**97**(7):657–62.

79. Mueller R, Petty T, Filley G. Ventilation and arterial blood gas exchange produced by pursed-lips breathing. *J Appl Physiol* 1970;**28**:784–9.

80. Tiep BL, Burns M, Kao D, et al. Pursed lips breathing training using ear oximetry. *Chest* 1986;**90**:218–21.

81. Puente-Maetsu L, Stringer W. Hyperinflation and its management in COPD. *Int J COPD* 2006;**1**(4):381–400.

82. Breslin EH. The pattern of respiratory muscle recruitment during pursed-lip breathing. *Chest* 1992;**101**:75–8.

83. Thoman RL, Stroker GL, Ross JC. The efficacy of pursed-lips breathing in patients with chronic obstructive pulmonary disease. *Am Rev Resp Dis* 1966;**93**:100–6.

84. Stockley RA, O'Brien C, Pye A, Hill SL. Relationship of sputum color to nature and outpatient management of acute exacerbations of COPD. *Chest* 2000;**117**(6):1638–45.

85. Pien GW, Pack AI. Chapter 79: Sleep disordered breathing. In: Mason RJ, et al., editors. *Murray and Nadel's Textbook of Respiratory Medicine*. 5th ed. Philadelphia: Saunders/Elsevier; 2010.

86. Johnson A. Sputum color: potential implications for clinical practice. *Respir Care* 2008;**53**(4):450.

87. Morris CG, Safranek S, Neher J. Clinical inquiries. Is sputum evaluation useful for patients with community-acquired pneumonia? *J Fam Pract* 2005;**54**(3):279–81.

88. Anevlavisa S, Petrogloub N, Tzavarasb A, et al. A prospective study of the diagnostic utility of sputum Gram stain in pneumonia. *J Infect* 2009;**59**(2):83–9.

89. Mancuso RF. Stridor in neonates. *Pediatr Clin North Am* 1996;**43**(6):1339–56.

90. Holinger LD. Etiology of stridor in the neonate, infant and child. *Ann Otol Rhinol Laryngol* 1980;**89**:397–400.

91. Grundfast KM, Harley EH. Vocal cord paralysis. *Otolaryngol Clin North Am* 1989;**22**:569–97.

92. Richardson MA, Cotton RT. Anatomic abnormalities of the pediatric airway. *Pediatr Clin North Am* 1984;**31**:821–34.

93. Ferguson CF. Congenital abnormalities of the infant larynx. *Ann Otol Rhinol Laryngol* 1967;**76**:744–52.

94. Cheng AC, Black JF, Buising KL. Respiratory rate the neglected sign: letter to editor. *Med J Aust* 2008;**189**(9):531.

95. Fieselmann JF, Hendry MS, Helms CM, Wakefield DS. Respiratory rate predicts cardiopulmonary arrest for internal medicine inpatients. *J Gen Intern Med* 1993;**8**(7):354–60.

96. Subbe CP, Davies RG, Williams E, et al. Effect of introducing the Modified Early Warning score on clinical outcomes, cardio-pulmonary arrests and intensive care utilisation in acute medical admissions. *Anaesthesia* 2003;**58**:797–802.

97. Goldhill DR, McNarry AF, Mandersloot G, et al. A physiologically-based early warning score for ward patients: the association between score and outcome. *Anaesthesia* 2005;**60**:547–53.

98. Cretikos M, Chen J, Hillman K, et al. The Objective Medical Emergency Team Activation Criteria: a case–control study. *Resuscitation* 2007;**73**:62–72.

99. Fujita MS, Tambara K, Budgell MS, Miyamoto S, Tambara K, Budgell B. Trepopnea in patients with chronic heart failure. *Int J Cardiol* 2002;**84**:115–18.

100. Schneider de Araujo B. Trepopnea may explain right-sided pleural effusion in patients with decompensated heart failure. *Am J Emerg Med* 2012;**30**(6):925–31.

101. Buller AJ, Dornhorst AC. The physics of some pulmonary sounds. *Lancet* 1956;**2**:649–52.

102. Baughman RP, Loudon RG. Sound spectral analysis of voice transmitted sound. *Am Rev Respir Dis* 1986;**134**:167–9.

103. Earis J. Lung sounds. *Thorax* 1992;**47**:671–2.

104. Marini JJ, Pierson DJ, Hudson LD, Lakshminarayan S. The significance of wheeze in chronic airflow obstruction. *Am Rev Respir Dis* 1979;**120**:1069–72.

105. Baughman RP, Loudon RG. Quantitation of wheezing in acute asthma. *Chest* 1984;**86**(5):718–22.

106. Bentur L. Wheeze monitoring in children for assessment of nocturnal asthma and response to therapy. *Eur Respir J* 2003;**21**(4):621–6.

1

CHAPTER 2

CARDIOVASCULAR SIGNS

Apex beat (also cardiac impulse)

Description

The normal cardiac impulse or 'apex beat' should be felt in the left fifth intercostal space in the midclavicular line over an area 2–3 cm^2 in diameter.[1]

The normal impulse is described as a brief outward thrust occurring in early systole and will disappear before S2 is heard. It coincides with isovolumetric contraction.

CLINICAL PEARL

Arterial pulse

The arterial pulse waveform can be difficult to classify and is an often-neglected clinical sign. The differences between pulse patterns may be subtle and therefore difficult (or impossible) for the expert as well as the novice to detect clinically without intra-arterial monitoring. They are discussed as a group for ease of comparison, and the important clinical pulse forms are highlighted. In order to understand the mechanism/s that create alternative pulse waveforms and the differences between them, a basic revision of the normal arterial waveform and some important definitions are first explained.

Key concept explained
The normal arterial waveform

Like the jugular venous pulse, the arterial pulse has a waveform, as shown in Figure 2.1. The waveform and arterial pressure are made up of two main components: the *pulse wave* (or pressure wave) and the *wave reflection*.

Pulse wave
The pulse wave is the pressure felt against the finger when palpating a pulse and represents the wave produced by left ventricular contraction.

Wave reflection
The waveform felt when taking a pulse, which is visible on monitoring, is created by more than just the pulse wave or forward flow of systole. Narrowing and bifurcation of blood vessels cause impedance, which forces the pressure wave to be reflected back on itself, and the systolic blood pressure and waveform to be amplified. The easiest analogy to use is that of waves in the ocean: if one wave travelling in one direction hits another wave heading in the opposite direction, the resulting collision is larger than the two independent waves.[2]

Anacrotic limb or upstroke
The anacrotic or ascending limb of the arterial waveform mainly reflects the pressure pulse produced by left ventricular contraction.[3]

Dicrotic limb and dicrotic notch
The dicrotic or descending limb of the waveform represents the decreasing pressure after left ventricular contraction. The dicrotic notch represents the closure of the aortic valve and retrograde or regurgitant flow across the valve.

Arterial pulse

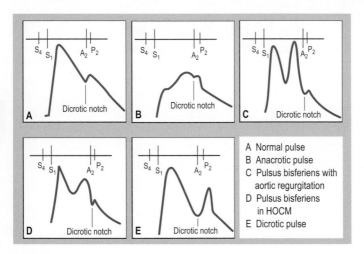

FIGURE 2.1
Configurational changes of the carotid pulse

A Normal pulse; **B** anacrotic pulse; **C** pulsus bisferiens; **D** pulsus bisferiens; **E** dicrotic pulse.

Based on Chatterjee K, Bedside evaluation of the heart: the physical examination. In: Chatterjee K et al. (eds), Cardiology. An Illustrated Text/Reference, *Philadelphia: JB Lippincott, 1991: Fig 48.5.*

Important concept explained
The Venturi principle

The Venturi principle is central to understanding the mechanism of arterial pulse signs. It states that when fluid flows through a constricted pipe (in this case a blood vessel), the pressure of the fluid (blood) drops. This causes constriction of the vessel (see Figure 2.2).

The importance of this will be demonstrated in the clinical signs following.

TABLE 2.1
Summary of pulse types

Pulse name	Key features	Condition/s
Alternans	Alternating strong and weak beats	Advanced left ventricular failure
Anacrotic	Slow rising, late peaking, interrupted upstroke	Aortic stenosis
Bigeminal	Two pulses in rapid succession then long pause	Severe heart failure Hypovolaemia Sepsis Benign
Bisferiens	2 beats per cardiac cycle – BOTH in systole. Accentuated notch	Aortic regurgitation HOCM
Dicrotic	2 beats per cardiac cycle one in systole, one in diastole	Myocardial dysfunction or low stroke volumes WITH intact systemic resistance
Pulsus parvus et tardus	Low amplitude and late peaking	Aortic stenosis
Pulus paradoxus		Cardiac tamponade Severe asthma

Venturi principle

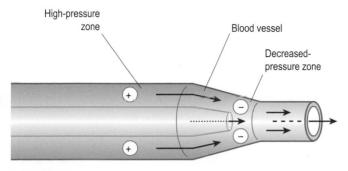

FIGURE 2.2
Schematic representation of the Venturi principle

Based on Vender JS, Clemency MV, Oxygen delivery systems, inhalation therapy, and respiratory care. In: Benumof JL (ed), Clinical Procedures in Anesthesia and Intensive Care, *Philadelphia: JB Lippincott, 1992: Fig 13-3.*

Bradycardia

Description

A heart rate of less than 60 beats per minute.

Condition/s associated with

The individual causes of bradycardia are too numerous to list. They include, but are not limited to:

More common

- Myocardial infarction
- Sinus node disease
- Drugs (e.g. beta blockers, calcium channel blockers, amiodarone)
- Hypothyroidism
- AV nodal disease
- Heart block
- Degeneration/ageing of the heart

Less common

- Cellular hypoxia
- Myocarditis
- Electrolyte imbalances
- Inflammatory disease (e.g. SLE)
- Obstructive sleep apnoea
- Haemochromatosis
- Congenital defect

Mechanism/s

The individual mechanisms for each underlying cause of bradycardia are numerous. In terms of a final common pathway, bradycardia is caused by:

- an interruption to or blocking of the conduction of electrical impulses in the heart

or

- an increase in vagal tone to the heart.

The disturbance can be present at the SA node, AV node, bundle of His or left or right bundle branches.

Myocardial infarction

May cause heart block, particularly if the right coronary artery (which feeds the AV and SA nodes in the majority of people) is occluded. Failure to deliver blood to the nodes causes ischaemia and, thus, SA and AV node dysfunction.

Cellular hypoxia

Decrease in oxygen from any cause (although usually ischaemic) can cause depolarisation of the SA node membrane potential, causing bradycardia; severe hypoxia completely stops pacemaker activity.

Sinus node disease

Damage to or degeneration of the sinus node leads to a number of problems, such as discharging at an irregular rate or pauses or discharges with subsequent blockage. All of these irregularities may cause bradycardia.

Heart block

Damage or disruption at the atria, AV node, bundle of His or in the bundle branches may slow conduction around the heart and cause heart block.

Electrolyte imbalances

Potassium, in particular, influences the membrane activity of cardiac myocytes as well as the SA and AV nodes. Significant variations in potassium concentration will affect membrane polarisation and heart rate. Bradycardia is more associated with hyperkalaemia than hypokalaemia, although it may be present with either.

Haemochromatosis

Iron infiltration that damages both the myocytes and conduction system of the heart has been shown to cause bradycardia.

Drugs

Drugs act by a variety of mechanisms to precipitate bradycardia:

- Calcium channel blockers inhibit the slow inward Ca^{+2} currents during SA node action potentials.
- Beta blockers and muscarinics act directly at the autonomic receptors, blocking sympathetic activity or enhancing parasympathetic activity.
- Digoxin enhances vagal tone to the AV node, slowing the heart rate.

Sign value

With so many potential causes of bradycardia, the specificity of the sign for a given disease is low. However, if noted in a patient who should otherwise have a normal heart rate, it warrants immediate attention.

Capillary return decreased/ delayed

Description

The time taken for a distal capillary bed to regain normal colour after sufficient pressure has been applied to cause blanching.[4] Delayed capillary return is usually described as a return to normal colour which takes longer than 2–3 seconds.

Condition/s associated with

- Dehydration
- Hypovolaemia
- Peripheral vascular disease
- Decreased peripheral perfusion (e.g. heart failure)

Mechanism/s

The normal components of peripheral perfusion are complex. Normal capillary perfusion is based on the driving pressure, arteriolar tone, capillary patency and density.[4] These, in turn, are influenced by a number of factors such as noradrenaline, angiotensin II, vasopression, endothelin 1 and thromboxane A2, all of which cause arteriolar vasoconstriction and may decrease capillary return, whereas prostacyclin, nitric oxide and local metabolites all may produce vasodilatation and increase capillary return. The interplay between these elements is thought to alter the ability of the blood to refill post blanching. There is limited scientific evidence to support this theory.[4]

Dehydration mechanism/s

In dehydration, the body's compensatory system tries to redistribute available fluid from the periphery to the central vasculature to maintain preload and, ultimately, cardiac output. The sympathetic nervous system is also invoked, resulting in peripheral vasoconstriction via local and neurohormonal mechanisms. This leads to decreased peripheral perfusion of the distal capillary beds and decreased or delayed capillary return.

Decreased peripheral perfusion mechanism/s

In heart failure, there is a lack of forward flow or 'driving pressure' to perfuse the distal capillary beds effectively. The body also compensates for poor forward flow by activating the sympathetic nervous system, the renin–angiotensin system, vasopressin and other factors that increase arteriolar tone, cause vasoconstriction and alter the time for distal capillary beds to refill.

Shocked state mechanism/s

In 'shocked' states (particularly sepsis), it is thought that an imbalance between vasoconstrictor and vasodilator substances and endothelial dysfunction occurs with the result that normal regulation of microvascular blood flow is impaired.[4]

Other factors, including arteriovenous shunting, 'no flow' capillaries, intermittent flow capillaries, increased capillary permeability and interstitial oedema, as well as leukocyte- and red-blood-cell-derived thrombi, may decrease functional capillary density and capillary refill.[4]

Sign value

As a sign, capillary refill or return suffers from significant inter-rater variability. Additionally, factors such as temperature and age can vary the time for refilling without pathology being present. Evidence is more robust in children (where it is used frequently) and is still very useful in adults if obviously deranged.

- One study found a capillary refill time (CRT) of >3 seconds suggests a fluid deficit greater than 100ml/kg in paediatric patients.[5]

- One systematic review found CRT was one of the strongest warning signs for serious paediatric infections in developed countries.[6]

- A review of studies including 478 patients found capillary refill time as the most useful individual sign for predicting 5% dehydration in children with a PLR of 4.1 with sensitivity 60% and specificity 85%.[7]

2

Cheyne–Stokes breathing

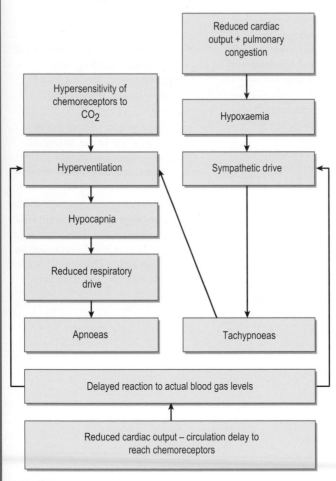

FIGURE 2.3
Flow diagram of Cheyne–Stokes respiration

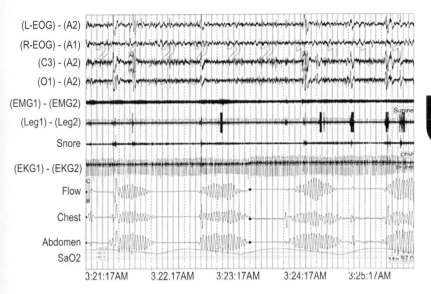

FIGURE 2.4
Polysomnogram of a patient with Cheyne-Stokes respiration. Note the periods of airflow and chest movement and then periods of apnoea

Description

Cheyne–Stokes respiration is technically described as a breathing pattern characterised by alternating apnoeas and tachypnoeas with a crescendo–decrescendo pattern of tidal volume. In practice, what will be seen is a rhythmic waxing and waning of the depth of respiration. The patient breathes deeply for a short time and then breathes very shallowly or stops breathing altogether.[8] The clinical sign can also be depicted on a polysomnogram seen in Figure 2.4. When looking at the flow, in the chest and abdomen leads there is rhythmic movement, followed by an apnoea.

Condition/s associated with

More common

- Congestive heart failure[8]
- Stroke

Less common

- Traumatic brain injury
- Brain tumours
- Carbon monoxide poisoning
- Morphine administration

Mechanism/s

Underlying damage or changes to the brainstem respiratory centre (which is responsible for involuntary respiration).

Mechanism/s in congestive heart failure

Several metabolic changes that affect chemoreceptors, the autonomic nervous system and the brainstem have been identified:

- Hypersensitivity of central chemoreceptors in the brainstem to changes in arterial blood carbon dioxide levels can lead to hyperventilation. This 'blowing off' causes a significant drop in carbon dioxide levels resulting in a central apnoea[9,10] (i.e. a drop in respiratory drive). The apnoea allows carbon dioxide to accumulate, stimulate respiratory drive and start the cycle again.

- Hypoxaemia due to lowered cardiac output and pulmonary congestion induces hyperventilation, leading to hypocapnia and an apnoea.[11]

- Hypoxaemia and hypercapnia combine to increase the sensitivity of the central breathing centre and cause an imbalance in respiration.[12]

- Heart enlargement and pulmonary congestion reduce pulmonary reservoirs of oxygen and carbon dioxide, especially during sleep, making the respiratory cycle more variable and less stable.

- With circulation delay, decreased cardiac output means it takes longer for oxygenated blood to reach peripheral chemoreceptors and help regulate ventilation. In contrast, the respiratory centre in the medulla can sense changes in pH and stimulate respiration to lower carbon dioxide immediately via the nervous system. The relatively slow feedback system of circulation means that changes to blood gas concentrations are often delayed and not truly representative,[11] causing an under- or over-activation of respiration and an ineffective feedback system to ventilatory regulation in the medulla.

- Increased levels of adrenaline have been seen in patients with CHF[12] due to over-activation of the sympathetic nervous system. Adrenaline increases minute ventilation, thus potentially increasing the 'blowing off' of carbon dioxide, causing hypocapnia and apnoea.

Sign value

A valuable sign, Cheyne–Stokes breathing is common in patients with an ejection fraction of less than 40%[12] and is seen in 50% of patients with CHF.[11] Studies have shown that patients with heart failure who experience Cheyne–Stokes breathing have a worse prognosis than those who do not.

Clubbing

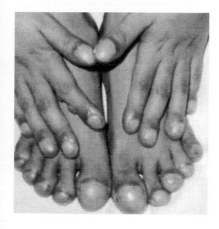

FIGURE 2.5
Clubbing of fingers and toes

Reproduced, with permission, from Marx JA, Hockberger RS, Walls RM et al. (eds), Rosen's Emergency Medicine, 7th edn, Philadelphia: Mosby, 2009: Fig 29.2.

Description

A characteristic bulging of the distal finger and nail bed, often described in stages:

1 Softening of the nail bed, causing a spongy feeling when the nail is pressed
2 Loss of the normal <165° angle between nail bed and fold
3 Convex nail growth
4 Thickening of the distal part of the finger
5 Shine and striation of the nail and skin

Condition/s associated with

Clubbing has a large number of differential diagnoses. The vast majority of clubbing is bilateral. Unilateral clubbing is very rare and has been seen in patients with hemiplegia, dialysis fistulas and ulnar artery AV malformations.

Pulmonary and neoplastic causes are by far the most common causes (see Table 2.2).

Mechanism/s

Many theories have been developed that attempt to explain clubbing; however, the mechanism for each aetiology is still unclear. Vasodilatation and proliferation of the distal nail beds is thought to be key and has been demonstrated in small MRI studies;[13] however, why vasodilatation occurs and what other contributing elements are present is not known. The lungs are thought to play a role in stopping factors that may precipitate clubbing from reaching the distal circulation. This theory is supported by observation that patients with untreated patent ductus arteriosus (PDA) demonstrate clubbing that is confined to the feet. The PDA is thought to provide an avenue for blood from the pulmonary artery which bypasses the lungs and is shunted into the descending aorta.

2

TABLE 2.2
Causes of bilateral clubbing

Neoplastic	Pulmonary
Bronchogenic carcinoma	Cystic fibrosis
Lymphoma	Asbestosis
Pleural tumours	Pulmonary fibrosis
	Sarcoidosis
	Hypertrophic pulmonary osteoarthropathy (HPOA)
Cardiac	**Gastrointestinal**
Cyanotic heart disease	Inflammatory bowel disease
Endocarditis	Liver disease
	Coeliac disease
Infectious	**Endocrinological**
Tuberculosis	Thyroid disease
Infective endocarditis	
HIV	

The most currently accepted explanation involves *platelets and platelet-derived growth factor (PDGF)*.[14] This theory does not explain unilateral clubbing and is not applicable to all cases where clubbing is present.

It is hypothesised that in healthy individuals, megakaryocytes are broken down into fragments in the lungs and these fragments become platelets. If this fragmentation does not occur, whole megakaryocytes can become wedged in the small vessels of distal extremities. Once trapped, they release PDGFs, which recruit cells and promote proliferation of muscle cells and fibroblasts. This cell proliferation causes the characteristic appearance of clubbing.

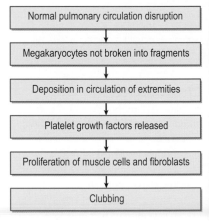

FIGURE 2.6
Proposed mechanism of clubbing

Therefore, any pathology that affects normal pulmonary circulation (such as cardiac shunts or lung disease) may allow whole megakaryocytes to enter the peripheral circulation unfragmented.

In bowel disease, it is suggested that the polycythaemia and arteriovenous malformations of the lung seen in some instances contribute to this process. In addition, vascular endothelial growth factor (VEGF) has been isolated in some patients with lung cancer and hypertrophic pulmonary osteoarthropathy (HPOA) and is likely to contribute to hyperplasia of the distal digits.

Sign value
Clubbing is almost always pathological and should be investigated; however, its absence does not exclude underlying disease.

2

Crackles (also rales)

Description

Popping, crackling, rattling or clicking sounds heard on lung auscultation that may be inspiratory or expiratory in timing.

Condition/s associated with

More common

- Left heart failure/pulmonary oedema – classically mid- to end-inspiratory
- Pneumonia
- Atelectasis
- Bronchiectasis
- Bronchitis
- Interstitial lung disease

Mechanism/s

Heart failure

In left heart failure, raised left ventricular and atrial pressures back up into the lung vasculature. When pulmonary vasculature pressure increases above 19mm Hg, a transudate of fluid enters the lung interstitium and alveoli. The alveoli are filled with fluid and collapse. When the patient breathes in, the alveoli are filled with air and 'pop' open, causing inspiratory crackles.

Other

Accumulation of phlegm, debris, mucus, blood or pus in the alveoli or small airways as a result of

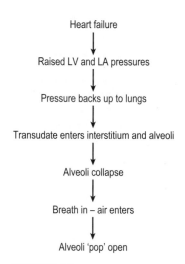

FIGURE 2.7
Mechanism of crackles in heart failure

pneumonia, haemoptysis, inflammatory disorder or any other aetiology will cause the alveoli to collapse and then potentially be 'popped' open, creating crackles.

Sign value

Crackles or rales are the most common sign in acute heart failure – seen in up to 66–87% of patients.[15,16] In the setting of acute heart failure without concomitant lung pathology, crackles are highly specific for heart failure. They are less valuable in chronic heart failure as the compensatory increased lymphatic drainage will shift fluid away more effectively.

Cyanosis

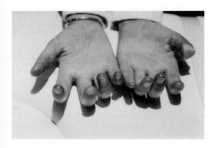

FIGURE 2.8
Photograph of hands of a 22-year-old female patient with SLE of 2 years duration
Extreme peripheral vasospasm and cyanosis was associated with early terminal gangrene in the right thumb (bandaged) and later several other digits.

Williams RC, Autoimmune disease etiology – a perplexing paradox or a turning leaf? Autoimmun Rev 2007-03-01Z, 6(4): 204–208, Fig 2. Copyright © 2006.

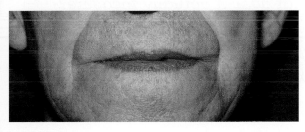

FIGURE 2.9
Central cyanosis of the lips

Douglas G, Nicol F, Robertson C, Macleod's Clinical Examination, 13th edn, Churchill Livingstone, Fig 3.6. Copyright © 2013.

Jugular venous pressure (JVP)

The signs associated with jugular venous pressure (JVP) are some of the first and most useful to be introduced to students studying cardiology. Jugular venous pressure is still the cornerstone of bedside assessment of volume/left ventricular filling pressure. It is integral to diagnostic and management decisions even while other more sophisticated tests are undertaken.

Key concept explained
JVP what does it actually measure?

When casting a knowing look at the internal jugular vein (and sometimes the external jugular vein), both of which drain via the superior vena cava into the right atrium, the clinician is using its features to estimate central venous pressure (CVP). CVP refers to right atrial pressure and, providing there is no tricuspid stenosis, right ventricular diastolic pressure.

This in turn is influenced by parts of the circuit seen in Figure 2.10.

These include the blood volume itself, the right ventricle, the pulmonary artery, the lungs, the pulmonary veins and the left side of the heart. Changes or dysfunction along this circuit at any point may cause changes to the JVP. For example, a decrease in circulating blood volume such as occurs in dehydration, may cause the JVP to be low, whereas a decrease in compliance due to infarction of the right ventricle will lead to decreased relaxation of the right ventricle and increased pressure for the given volume, and therefore a higher jugular venous pressure. Understanding the flow and circuit in Figure 2.10 is crucial in understanding the different causes of change to the JVP.

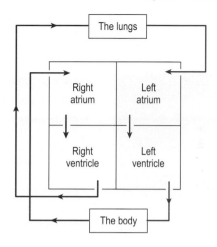

FIGURE 2.10
Stylised diagram of the pulmonary and systemic circuits
Interruptions or changes in pressure along the circuits cause changes in pressure
upstream of the underlying pathology.

Peripheral oedema

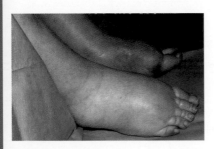

FIGURE 2.11
Peripheral oedema

Rangaprasad L et al., Itraconazole associated quadriparesis and edema: a case report. Journal of Medical Case Reports *2011; 5: 140.*

Definition

An abnormal accumulation of fluid under the skin or within body cavities, causing swelling of the area or indentations on firm palpation.

Condition/s associated with

Diseases associated with peripheral oedema are numerous. Main causes include:

More common

- Congestive cardiac failure
- Liver disease
- Nephrotic syndrome
- Renal failure
- Venous insufficiency
- Drug side effects
- Pregnancy

Less common

- Hypoalbuminaemia
- Malignancy

Mechanism/s

The mechanism underlying peripheral oedema is dependent on the underlying pathology. However, regardless of aetiology, either one or a combination of the following factors is present:

1 increased venous or hydrostatic pressure – raising capillary hydrostatic pressure (increased pressure pushing fluid out)

2 reduced interstitial hydrostatic pressure (reduced pressure pushing fluid into vessels)

3 decreased plasma oncotic pressure (decreased proteins keeping fluid in the vessel)

4 increased interstitial oncotic pressure (increased proteins trying to draw fluid out of vessels)

5 increased capillary leakiness

6 blocked lymphatic system – decreased ability to draw fluid and proteins away from interstitium and return them to the normal circulation.

Mechanism in heart failure

Increased venous hydrostatic pressure causes a transudative process in which fluid is 'pushed out' of vessels into the interstitium. It is normally seen in the context of *right* heart failure.

Factors contributing to this include:

- *Increased plasma volume* – decreased cardiac output (either via right or left heart failure) leads to renal hypoperfusion. In response to this, the RAAS is activated and salt and water are retained, leading to increased venous and capillary hydrostatic pressure.

- *Raised venous pressure* – ventricular dysfunction leads to increased end-systolic and/or end-diastolic pressures – these pressures are transmitted back to the atrium and then to the venous system, increasing venous and capillary hydrostatic pressure.

- Increased hydrostatic pressure forces fluid out of venous vessels into surrounding tissues.

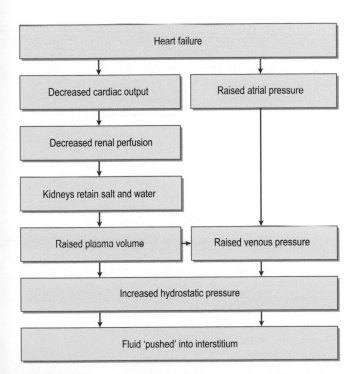

FIGURE 2.12
Peripheral oedema in heart failure

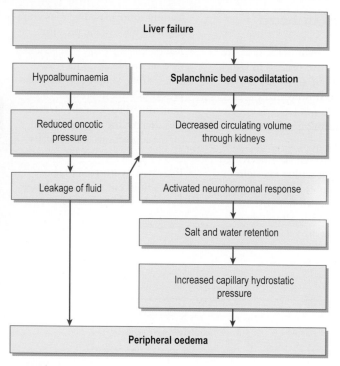

FIGURE 2.13
Peripheral oedema in liver failure

- The lymphatic system is unable to keep up with the task of reabsorbing additional interstitial fluid and oedema develops.

Liver disease

Contrary to popular belief, the main factor in the development of oedema in liver failure is *vasodilatation of the splanchnic bed*. It is not necessarily a consequence of the liver failing to produce its normal proteins (leading to hypoalbuminaemia), although this may contribute.

In liver failure, increased nitric oxide and prostaglandins are present in the splanchnic circulation. This vasodilates the splanchnic vessels, leading to more blood being 'pooled' there, with less effective circulating volume driven through the kidneys, leading to an aberrant neurohormonal response that results in increased salt and water retention through the RAAS, increasing hydrostatic pressure.[17]

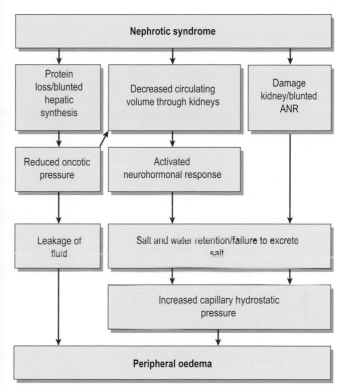

FIGURE 2.14
Peripheral oedema in nephrotic syndrome

Nephrotic syndrome

The mechanism of oedema in nephrotic syndrome has not been completely worked out. Factors involved include:

- Massive protein loss through the kidneys and hypoalbuminaemia, decreased plasma oncotic pressure (i.e. there are fewer proteins keeping fluid in) so fluid leaks out.

- Loss of circulating volume triggers a neurohormonal response with increased salt and water retention, increasing capillary hydrostatic pressure – pushing fluid out.

- Blunted hepatic protein synthesis contributes to the low quantity of proteins in the serum.

- Blunted atrial natriuretic response (ANR) – the normal response to volume overload is to excrete more salt and thus water out via the kidneys.

- The renal impairment seen in nephrotic and nephritic syndromes does not allow the 'normal' amount of salt to be excreted, thus fluid is retained. This is possibly the predominant mechanism in the absence of massive protein loss.[17]

Sign value

Peripheral oedema is a useful sign when present; however, its absence does not exclude heart failure (sensitivity 10%, specificity 93%[18]) with only 25% of patients with chronic heart failure under 70 years of age having oedema.

In liver failure, the development of peripheral oedema, and in particular ascites, heralds a poor prognosis.

Skin turgor: decreased

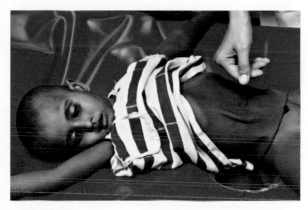

FIGURE 2.15
A child with cholera showing decreased skin turgor
From Sack DA, Sack RB, Nair GB, et al., Cholera, Lancet 2004; 363: 223–233.

Description
A decrease in skin turgor is indicated when the skin (on the back of the hand for an adult or on the abdomen for a child) is gently pinched for a few seconds and does not return to its original state when released.

Condition/s associated with
- Age
- Dehydration
- Ehlers–Danlos syndrome

Mechanism/s
Normal skin elasticity or turgor is dependent on collagen, elastin and fluid content. In dehydrated patients, available fluid and water in the body is reabsorbed and used to supplement circulating volume. Fluid from the skin is no exception. With decreased water in the layers of the skin, turgor is decreased.

Ehlers–Danlos syndrome mechanism

In Ehlers–Danlos syndrome, there is a genetic mutation resulting in abnormal collagen synthesis. In classical Ehlers–Danlos, the mutation causes an abnormal type V collagen, whereas other forms affect different types of collagen and the extracellular matrix. Collagen is essential for skin strength and elasticity and, therefore, defects in this can produce thin and elastic skin resulting in decreased skin turgor.

Sign value

The sign of poor skin turgor suffers from high interobserver variability. As skin turgor decreases with age the most robust evidence is with regard to children. In pooled studies of 602 patients across five studies, abnormal skin turgor was associated with 5% or greater dehydration in children 2–15 years, with a sensitivity of 58% (40–75 95% CI), specificity 76% (59–93 CI) with a PLR of 2.42.[7]

Tachycardia (sinus)

Description

A regular heart rate of more than 100 beats per minute.

Condition/s associated with

Sinus tachycardia is associated with a number of conditions. These may be normal physiological responses or a reaction to a pathological insult. The conditions include, but are not limited to:

More common

- Exercise
- Anxiety
- Pain
- Fever/infection
- Hypovolaemia
- Anaemia
- Decreased cardiac output (e.g. heart failure)
- Sino-atrial node dysfunction
- Pulmonary embolism
- Hyperthyroidism
- Stimulants and drugs (e.g. caffeine, beta-2 agonists, cocaine)
- Hypoxia
- Myocardial infarction

Less common

- Phaeochromocytoma

Mechanism/s

Knowing the mechanism for each cause of tachycardia is impractical. For most causes the final common pathway for the development of sinus tachycardia is activation of the sympathetic nervous system and/or catecholamine release. This can be appropriate in the case of anxiety, fear or hypovolaemia, or inappropriate in the case of a phaeochromocytoma or drugs that release (or cause the release of) catecholamines.

Mechanism in hyperthyroidism

The mechanism of tachycardia in hyperthyroidism is unique and is a result of *increased T3 levels*.

T3 has genomic (induction and expression of specific genes) and non–genomic properties that influence the production and alter the performance of myofibrillary proteins, sarcoplasmic reticula, ATPases and sodium, potassium and calcium channels. The end result is increased contractility and increased heart rate and cardiac output.[19]

2

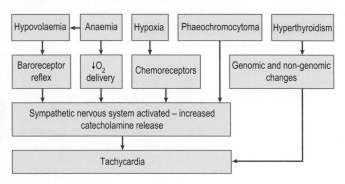

FIGURE 2.16
Mechanisms of tachycardia

Sign value

Isolated tachycardia is a very non-specific sign. Its value as a clinical sign is dependent on context. However, studies have shown the following:

- It has limited independent value in predicting hypovolaemia.[20]

- In conjunction with other variables, it has value in predicting pneumonia.[21]

- In trauma, sepsis pneumonia and myocardial infarction, tachycardia has been shown to have prognostic value in predicting increased risk of mortality.[22–26]

References

1. Karnath B, Thornton W. Precordial and carotid pulse palpation. *Hosp Physician* 2002;20–4.

2. Vlachopoulos C, O'Rourke M. Genesis of the normal and abnormal arterial pulse. *Curr Probl Cardiol* 2000;**25**(5):300–67.

3. McGhee BH, Bridges MEJ. Monitoring arterial blood pressure: what you may not know. *Crit Care Nurse* 2002;**22**:60–79.

4. Pickard A, et al. Capillary refill time: is it still a useful clinical sign? *Anesth Analg* 2011;**113**(1):120–3.

5. Saavedra JM, et al. Capillary refilling (skin turgor) in the assessment of dehydration. *Am J Dis Child* 1991;**145**:296–8.

6. Van den Bruel A, Haj-Hassan T, Thompson M, Butinx F, Mant D. Diagnostic value of clinical features at presentation to identify serious infection in children in developed countries: a systematic review. *Lancet* 2010;**375**:135–42.

7. Steiner MJ, et al. Is this child dehydrated? *JAMA* 2004;**291**(22):2746–854.

8. Dorland WAN. *Dorland's Illustrated Medical Dictionary*, 30th ed. Philadelphia: Saunders; 2003.

9. Javaheri S. A mechanism of central sleep apnoea in patients in heart failure. *N Engl J Med* 1999;**341**:949–54.

10. Wilcox I, Grunstein RR, Collins FL, Berthon-Jones M, Kelly DT, Sullivan CE. The role of central chemosensitivity in central sleep apnoea of heart failure. *Sleep* 1993;**16**:S37–8.

11. Ingbir M, Freimark D, Motro M, Adler Y. The incidence, pathophysiology, treatment and prognosis of Cheyne–Stokes breathing disorder in patients with congestive heart failure. *Herz* 2002;**2**:107–12.

12. Yoshiro Y, Kryger MH. Sleep in heart failure. *Sleep* 1993;**16**:513–23.

13. Nakamura J, Halliday NA, Fukuba E, et al. The microanatomic basis of finger clubbing – a high-resolution magnetic resonance imaging study. *J Rheumatol* 2014; **41**(3):523–7.

14. Spicknall KE, Zirwas MJ, English JC. Clubbing: an update on diagnosis, differential diagnosis, pathophysiology and clinical relevance. *J Am Acad Dermatol* 2005;**52**:1020–8.

15. Tavazzi L, Maggioni AP, Lucci D, et al. Nationwide survey on acute heart failure in cardiology ward services in Italy. *Eur Heart J* 2006;**27**:1207–15.

16. ADHERE Scientific Advisory Committee: Acute Decompensated Heart Failure National Registry (ADHERE®). Core Module Q1 2006 Final Cumulative National Benchmark Report. Scios, Inc, 2006.

17. Schroth BE. Evaluation and management of peripheral edema. *JAAPA* 2005;**18**(11): 29–34.

18. William D, et al. *Heart Failure: A Comprehensive Guide to Diagnosis and Treatment*. New York: Marcel Dekker; 2005.

19. Klein I, Ojama K. Thyroid hormone and the cardiovascular system. *N Engl J Med* 2001;**344**(7):501–8.

20. Brasel KJ, Guse C, Gentilello LM, Nirula R. The heart rate: is it truly a vital sign? *Journal of Trauma – Injury, Infection, and Critical Care* 2007;**62**:812–17.

21. Heckerling PS, Tape TG, Wigton RS, et al. Clinical prediction rule for pulmonary infiltrates. *Ann Intern Med* 1990;**113**(9):664–770.

22. Victorino GP, Battistella FD, Wisner DH. Does tachycardia correlate with hypotension after trauma? *J Am Coll Surg* 2003;**196**:679–84.

23. Kovar D, Cannon CP, Bentley JH, et al. Does initial and delayed heart rate predict mortality in patients with acute coronary syndromes? *Clin Cardiol* 2004; **27**:80–6.

24. Zuanetti G, Mantini L, Hernandez-Bernal F, et al. Relevance of heart rate as a prognostic indicator in patients with acute myocardial infarction: insights from the GISSI 2 study. *Eur Heart J* 1998;**19**(Suppl. F):F19–26.

25. Leibovici L, Gafter-Gvili A, Paul M, et al. TREAT Study Group. Relative tachycardia in patients with sepsis: an independent risk factor for mortality. *QJM* 2007;**100**(10):629–34.

26. Parker MM, Shelhamer JH, Natanson C, Dalling DW, Parillo JE. Serial cardiovascular variables in survivors and nonsurvivors of human septic shock: heart rate as an early predictor of prognosis. *Crit Care Med* 1987;**15**:923–9.

CHAPTER 3

HAEMATOLOGICAL AND ONCOLOGICAL SIGNS

Ecchymoses, purpura and petechiae

Description

Ecchymoses, purpura and petechiae all refer to different sizes of subcutaneous haematomas. It is important to remember that any one condition can cause a range of stigmata. That is, a petechiae-causing

pathology may also produce ecchymoses. In reality, the origins will often overlap (see Table 3.1), and it is more important to have an understanding of the general mechanisms rather than the numerous disorders leading to them.

TABLE 3.1
Causes of petechiae, purpura and ecchymoses

Petechiae	Purpura	Ecchymoses
Description		
Small (1–2 mm) haemorrhages into mucosal or serosal surfaces	>3 mm haemorrhages, or when ecchymoses and petechiae form in groups[1]	Subcutaneous haematoma >10–20 mm
Condition/s associated with		
Thrombocytopenia of any cause (e.g. autoimmune, heparin-induced, hypersplenism) Bone marrow failure (e.g. malignancy) Defective platelet function (rare) (e.g. Glanzmann's thromboasthenia uraemia) Disseminated intravascular coagulation Infection Bone marrow defects Factor deficiencies	Diseases associated with: As for petechiae: • Trauma • Vasculitis – particularly *palpable* purpura • Amyloidosis • Over-anticoagulation • Factor deficiencies	As for petechiae and purpura: • Trauma – common Diseases causing: • Defective platelet action • Vasculitis – *palpable* purpura • Amyloidosis • Hereditary haemorrhagic telangiectasia • Scurvy • Cushing's syndrome • Over-anticoagulation • Factor deficiencies (e.g. haemophilia)

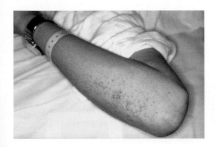

FIGURE 3.1
Petechiae in a patient with thrombocytopenia

Reproduced, with permission, from Little JW, Falace DA, Miller CS, Rhodus NL, Dental Management of the Medically Compromised Patient, 7th edn, St Louis: Mosby Elsevier, 2008: Fig 25-9.

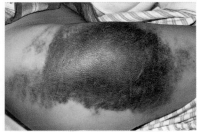

FIGURE 3.2
Ecchymoses in a patient with haemophilia

Reproduced, with permission, from Little JW, Falace DA, Miller CS, Rhodus NL, Dental Management of the Medically Compromised Patient, 7th edn, St Louis: Mosby Elsevier, 2008: Fig 25-16.

General mechanism/s

A subcutaneous haematoma of any size can be the result of a disruption of:

- the blood vessel wall
- the normal coagulation/clotting process
- the number or function of platelets.

The consequent subcutaneous bleeding (where haemoglobin produces the initial red/blue discolouration) can then be further classified by size.

Thrombocytopenia

A significant thrombocytopenia will result in inadequate control and clotting of any bleed. This is due to the lack of platelet activation and 'plugging'. Trauma from any cause, no matter how minor, may

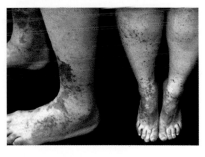

FIGURE 3.3
Palpable purpura
In a patient with Henoch–Schönlein purpura (left) and hepatitis C and cryoglobulinaemia (right).

Reproduced, with permission, from Libby P, Bonow R, Zipes R, Mann D, Braunwald's Heart Disease: A Textbook of Cardiovascular Medicine, 8th edn, Philadelphia: Saunders, 2007: Fig 84-1.

precipitate mucocutaneous bleeding and, without adequate clotting, petechiae, purpura or ecchymoses may develop before the bleed is controlled. It is rare to see spontaneous bleeding with thrombocytopenia until platelets are below $20\,000 \times 10^9$/L. Easy bruising can occur with minor trauma if platelets are between $20\,000 \times 10^9$/L and $50\,000 \times 10^9$/L.

Vasculitis
Inflammation of the small arterioles or venules in the skin, associated with immune complex deposition, produces inflammation with punctate oedema and haemorrhage and, thus, palpable purpura.[1]

Cushing's
Ecchymoses in Cushing's syndrome are related to a lack of connective tissue support in vessel walls, due to corticosteroid-induced reduction in collagen synthesis.[2]

Mechanism of colour changes
Once under the skin, erythrocytes are phagocytosed and degraded by macrophages, with haemoglobin converted to bilirubin, thus creating blue–green discolouration. Bilirubin is eventually broken down into haemosiderin (which is golden brown) at the end of the process before skin returns to its normal hue.

Sign value
Although there is limited evidence for the value of these lesions as clinical signs and the specificity is low, given the numerous potentially pathological causes, healthy patients rarely produce these signs and therefore they should be investigated if seen.

Lymphadenopathy

Description
Enlarged lymph nodes able to be palpated or identified on imaging.

Condition/s associated with
Numerous disorders can present with lymphadenopathy as part of their clinical picture. The acronym MIAMI may help the clinician recall the broad causes (see Table 3.2): **M**alignancy, **I**nfectious, **A**utoimmune, **M**iscellaneous and **I**atrogenic.[3]

General mechanism/s
In general, most of the conditions that result in lymphadenopathy do so either via:

1 propagation of an inflammatory response, whether it be systemic, regional or direct[4]
2 invasion and/or proliferation of abnormal or malignant cells.[4,5]

Malignancy
Malignancy causes lymphadenopathy through invasion or infiltration of malignant cells *into* the lymph node or direct proliferation of malignant cells *within* the lymph node.

The lymphatic system provides the predominant mechanism for distant metastatic spread of cells for a variety of solid-tumour cancers (e.g. colorectal, ovarian, prostate). Tumour cells move from the main tumour site via the lymphatic system to lymph nodes, where they accumulate and/or proliferate, enlarging the lymph node.

In lymphoma there is an abnormal proliferation of lymphocytes within the lymph node with associated hyperplasia of normal structures, producing lymphadenopathy.

Infectious causes
The lymphatic system is central to effective functioning of the immune system. Macrophages and other antigen-presenting cells migrate to the lymph nodes in order to present antigens to T and B cells. On recognition of an antigen, T and B cells proliferate within the lymph node in order to generate an effective immune response. The lymphadenopathy seen with infection (local or systemic) is a consequence of this proliferation.

Where *direct invasion* occurs, a solitary lymph node becomes infected with a bacterium or other type of antigen. The resulting immune response results in hyperplasia of the lymph node structures, T and B cell proliferation and infiltration of other immune cells to address the infection. This results in inflammation and swelling of the node.

In the presence of *systemic infection*, reactive hyperplasia can occur. An antigenic (intracellular or extracellular) stimulus is brought to

TABLE 3.2
Causes of lymphadenopathy – MIAMI acronym

M Malignancy	I Infectious	A Autoimmune	M Miscellaneous	I Iatrogenic
Lymphoma	Tonsillitis	Sarcoidosis	Kawasaki's disease	Serum sickness
Leukaemia	Epstein–Barr virus	SLE	Sarcoidosis	Drugs
Multiple myeloma	Tuberculosis	Rheumatoid arthritis		
Skin cancer	HIV			
Breast cancer	CMV			
	Streptococcal and staphylococcal infection			
	Cat scratch disease			

Based on McGee S, Evidence Based Physical Diagnosis, 2nd edn, Philadelphia: Saunders, 2007: Box 24.1; with permission.

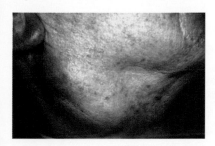

FIGURE 3.4
Cervical lymphadenopathy

Reproduced, with permission, from Little JW, Falace DA, Miller CS, Rhodus NL, Dental Management of the Medically Compromised Patient, *7th edn, St Louis: Mosby, 2008: Fig 24-6.*

TABLE 3.3
Values of lymph node characteristics in the diagnosis of malignancy or serious underlying disease

Feature	Value
Hard texture	Sensitivity 48–62%, specificity 83–84%, PLR 3.2, NLR 0.6
Fixed lymph nodes	Sensitivity 12–52%, specificity 97%, PLR 10.9
Lymph node size >9 cm²	Sensitivity 37–38%, specificity 91–98%, PLR 8.4

the lymph node and presented to T and B cells, lymphocytes and other cells resident in the node, causing their proliferation.[6]

Autoimmune

Autoimmune causes of lymphadenopathy are similar to infectious causes of lymphadenopathy, except that the antigen is a *self*-antigen and the *inflammatory response* is an *inappropriate* one. B cell proliferation is often seen within the lymph nodes of patients with rheumatoid arthritis whereas T cell proliferation is seen in systemic lupus erythematosus.[6]

Sign value

With so many potential causes for lymphadenopathy, its specificity as a sign is limited. The main issue for the clinician is to determine whether it is arising from a malignant cause or something more benign, such as infection.

Several characteristics are said to make a node more suggestive of malignancy. A review[7] of studies regarding these characteristics in the diagnosis of malignancy or serious underlying disease found that the features listed in Table 3.3 generally had higher specificity than sensitivity. That is, if the characteristic was present, it was suggestive of a serious underlying cause but, if it was not present, malignancy or another serious cause could not be ruled out. Evidence of supraclavicular lymphadenopathy is said to be more indicative of malignancy.

Time course of the development of lymphadenopathy is also used as an indicator of malignancy, with a shorter duration more likely due to an acute infective cause, and a longer time course suggestive of malignancy.

In one study of 457 children presenting with lymphadenopathy, in 98.2% of cases acute

Lymphadenopathy: location – location – location

The site of lymphadenopathy may help identify the origin of the underlying conditions. Detailed explanations of the anatomy of the lymph system can be found in any anatomy textbook. The drainage areas associated with various lymph nodes are given in brief in Table 3.4.

Using these anatomical landmarks, clinicians can narrow their search for the primary malignancy.

Generalised lymphadenopathy

Generalised lymphadenopathy is usually described as the enlargement of two or more groups of lymph nodes. It is caused by systemic disorders that by their nature affect more than just a localised region of the body. Such conditions include lymphoma, leukaemia, tuberculosis, HIV/AIDS, syphilis, other infectious diseases and some connective tissue disorders (e.g. rheumatoid arthritis). Although this principle is not absolute, it does help shorten the differential diagnosis list.

TABLE 3.4
Location of lymphadenopathy

Lymph node	Anatomical drainage area
Cervical	All of the head and neck
Supraclavicular	Thorax, abdominal organs (see Virchow's node)
Epitrochlear	Ulnar aspect or arm and hand[8]
Axillary	Ipsilateral arm, breast and chest
Inguinal – horizontal group	Lower anterior wall, lower anal canal
Inguinal – vertical group	Lower limb, penis, scrotum and gluteal area

lymphadenopathy was due to benign causes. Malignancies were most often associated with chronic and generalised lymphadenopathy.[9]

Painful versus painless nodes

It is generally believed that painful nodes are more likely to be reactive or related to an inflammatory process than painless nodes, which are more likely to be malignant. However, evidence for this assumption is limited.

3

Virchow's node – not just gastrointestinal malignancy

Virchow's node refers to supraclavicular lymphadenopathy and has classically been taught as a sign of gastrointestinal malignancy only, but recent research has shown broader associations.

Mechanism/s
Virchow's node is located at the end of the thoracic duct.[10] Accepted theory is that lymph and malignant cells from the gastrointestinal system travel through the thoracic duct and are deposited in Virchow's node.

Condition/s associated with
Studies[11] have now shown Virchow's node to be present with:
- lung cancer – most common[11]
- pancreatic cancer
- oesophageal cancer
- renal cancer
- ovarian cancer
- testicular cancer[12,13]
- stomach cancer
- prostate cancer
- uterine and cervical cancer
- gallbladder cancer – rare
- liver cancer
- adrenal cancer
- bladder cancer.

References

1. LeBlond RF, Brown DD, DeGowin RL. Chapter 6: The skin and nails. In: LeBlond RF, Brown DD, DeGowin RL, editors. *DeGowin's Diagnostic Examination*. 9th ed. Available: http://proxy14.use.hcn.com.au/content.aspx?aID=3659565 [2 Aug 2010].

2. Yanovski JA, Cutler GB Jr. Glucocorticoid action and the clinical features of Cushing's syndrome. *Endocrinol Metab Clin North Am* 1994;**23**:487–509.

3. Henry PH, Longo DL. Chapter 60: Enlargement of lymph nodes and spleen. In: Fauci AS, Braunwald E, Kasper DL, et al., editors. *Harrison's Principles of Internal Medicine*. 17th ed. Available: http://proxy14.use.hcn.com.au/content.aspx?aID=2875326 [18 Sep 2010].

4. LeBlond RF, Brown DD, DeGowin RL. Chapter 5: Non-regional systems and diseases. In: LeBlond RF, Brown DD, DeGowin RL, editors. *DeGowin's Diagnostic Examination*. 9th ed. Available: http://proxy14.use.hcn.com.au/content.aspx?aID=3659310. – lymphatic system [18 Sep 2010].

5. Bazemore AW, Smucker DR. Lymphadenopathy and malignancy. *Am Fam Phys* 2002;**66**(11):2103–10.

6. Jung W, Trumper L. Differential diagnosis and diagnostic strategies of lymphadenopathy. *Internist* 2008;**49**(3):305–18, quiz 319–20.

7. McGee S. *Evidence Based Physical Diagnosis*. 3rd ed. St Louis: Elsevier; 2012.

8. Selby CD, Marcus HS, Toghill PJ. Enlarged epitrochlear lymphnodes: an old sign revisited. *J R Coll Phys London* 1992;**26**(2):159–61.

9. Oguz A, Temel EA, Citak EC, Okur FV. Evaluation of peripheral lymphadenopathy in children. *Pediatr Hematol Oncol* 2006;**23**:549–51.

10. Mitzutani M, Nawata S, Hirai I, Murakami G, Kimura W. Anatomy and histology of Virchow's node. *Anat Sci Int* 2005;**80**:193–8.

11. Viacava EP. Significance of supraclavicular signal node in patients with abdominal and thoracic cancer. *Arch Surg* 1944;**48**:109–19.

12. Lee YTN, Gold RH. Localisation of occult testicular tumour with scrotal thermography. *JAMA* 1976;**236**:1975–6.

13. Slevin NJ, James PD, Morgan DAL. Germ cell tumours confined to the supraclavicular fossa: a report of two cases. *Eur J Surg Oncol* 1985;**11**:187–90.

CHAPTER 4

NEUROLOGICAL SIGNS

Understanding the clinical significance of neurological signs poses several challenges that require pre-requisite knowledge of:

- neuroanatomy and topographical anatomy (relevant adjacent structures)
- pathophysiology of neurological disorders and relevant adjacent structures
- pattern recognition of multiple clinical signs

Gag reflex

Relevant neuroanatomy and topographical anatomy[1-3]

CENTRAL PATHWAYS
- Vomiting centre, brainstem
- Cortical areas

AFFERENT LIMB – GLOSSOPHARYNGEAL NERVE (CNIX)
- ⊗ 'Trigger zones' – palatoglossal and palatopharyngeal folds, base of tongue, palate, uvula, posterior pharyngeal wall
  ↓
- Glossopharyngeal nerve fibres
  ↓
- Petrosal ganglion
- ⇒ Jugular foramen
  ↓
- Solitary nucleus, medulla
  ↓

EFFERENT LIMB – GLOSSOPHARYNGEAL NERVE (CNIX)
- Nucleus ambiguus, medulla
- ⇒ Jugular foramen
  ↓
- Petrosal ganglion
  ↓
- × Stylopharyngeus and superior pharyngeal constrictor muscles

EFFERENT LIMB – VAGUS NERVE (CNX)
- Nucleus ambiguus and dorsal motor nucleus, medulla
  ↓
- Vagus nerve
- ⇒ Jugular foramen
- ⇒ Nodose ganglion
  ↓
- × Palatal constrictors and intrinsic laryngeal muscles

4

Description

Absence of stylopharyngeus muscle and superior pharyngeal muscle constriction following stimulation of the posterior tongue and/or oropharynx.[1] Absence of the gag reflex can be unilateral or bilateral.

Condition/s associated with[1]

Common

- Normal variant
- Coma
- Drugs – ethanol, benzodiazepine, opioid
- Lateral medullary syndrome (Wallenberg's syndrome)

Less common

- Cerebellopontine tumour – acoustic schwannoma, glomus tumour
- Internal carotid artery dissection

Mechanism/s

The afferent limb of the gag reflex is mediated by the glossopharyngeal nerve (CNIX), whereas the efferent limb is mediated by the glossopharyngeal nerve (CNIX) and the vagus nerve (CNX).[1] External factors, such as nausea or chronic emesis, may confound the evaluation of the gag reflex, as they may sensitise or desensitise the gag response. Visual, auditory and olfactory stimuli may also sensitise the gag response.[4,5] The gag reflex is absent in a significant percentage of normal individuals.[6] Causes of an absent gag reflex include:

- normal variant
- generalised CNS depression
- glossopharyngeal nerve (CNIX) lesion
- vagus nerve (CNX) lesion
- lateral medullary syndrome (Wallenberg's syndrome).

Normal variant

The gag reflex is absent in a significant proportion of the population. Absence of the gag reflex is likely caused by suppression of the reflex by higher cortical centres and/or desensitisation of the reflex response with ageing.

Generalised CNS depression

The obtunded or comatose patient may have an absent gag reflex due to generalised central nervous system dysfunction.

Glossopharyngeal nerve lesion

Glossopharyngeal nerve palsy causes ispilateral loss of the gag reflex, decreased pharyngeal elevation, dysarthria and dysphagia.[1] Causes of glossopharygneal nerve dysfunction include cerebellopontine angle tumours, Chiari I malformations, jugular foramen syndrome, neoplasia and iatrogenic injury following laryngoscopy or tonsillectomy.[1]

Vagus nerve lesion

Vagus nerve dysfunction causes ipsilateral loss of pharyngeal and laryngeal sensation, unilateral loss of sensation in the external ear, dysphagia, hoarseness, unilateral paresis of the uvula and soft palate, and deviation of the uvula away from the side of the lesion.[1] Causes of vagus nerve dysfunction include internal carotid artery dissection, neoplasia and trauma.

Lateral medullary syndrome (Wallenberg's syndrome)

Lateral medullary syndrome most commonly results from posterior inferior cerebellar artery (PICA) territory infarction due to vertebral artery insufficiency. Infarction of the solitary nucleus and/or nucleus ambiguus in the medulla may result in an absent ipsilateral gag reflex.

Sign value

An absent gag reflex occurs in a significant percentage of the normal population. In a study of 140 healthy subjects at various ages, the gag reflex was absent in 37% of subjects.[6]

4

Photophobia

Relevant neuroanatomy and topographical anatomy

⇒ Cornea
⇒ Uvea

↓   ↓

- Non-image-forming retinal neuroepithelium
- Ophthalmic division (VI) trigeminal nerve (CNV) and C2, C3 sensory nerve cells, optic nerve
- Meninges

↓   ↓   ↓

- Region posterior thalamus, pain pathway

Description

Photophobia is light-induced ocular and/or cephalic discomfort.[7] The patient exhibits discomfort and aversion to light stimuli, resulting in involuntary eye closure and/or gaze deviation.

Condition/s associated with[7,8]

Common

- Migraine headache
- Corneal abrasion
- Keratitis – UV, contact lens

Less common

- Glaucoma
- Subarachnoid haemorrhage, aneurysmal
- Meningitis – bacterial, viral, fungal, aseptic
- Anterior uveitis
- HSV keratitis

Mechanism/s

The mechanism of photophobia is controversial.[7,9] Photophobia may be a protective mechanism that protects the central retina from potentially damaging short wavelength visible light.[7,9]

Causes of photophobia include:

- inflammation of the meninges
- migraine
- corneal injury
- anterior uveitis.

Inflammation of the meninges

Meningeal irritation is caused by infection, non-infectious inflammation, chemical inflammation and subarachnoid haemorrhage. Associated signs of meningeal irritation include nuchal rigidity, Kernig's sign, Brudzinski's sign and jolt accentuation.

Migraine

Non-image-forming retinal neuroepithelial cells project to an area in the posterior thalamus that also receives input from the dura mater. The cells in the posterior thalamus respond to input from both the non-image-forming retinal neuroepithelial cells and trigeminal and cervical nerves innervating the dura mater. In migraine, it has been suggested that input from the retinal neuroepithelial cells potentially augments migraine pain, resulting in photophobia.[9]

Corneal injury

Traumatic and inflammatory disorders of the cornea cause photophobia. The cornea is densely innervated, and light exacerbates ocular discomfort. Causes include contact lens acute red eye and corneal abrasion.

Anterior uveitis

Inflammation or mechanical irritation of the iris, pupillary sphincter muscle and radial muscle cause photophobia. Discomfort is likely exacerbated by mechanical stress due to the change in pupil size during the pupillary light response and hippus.[8]

Sign value

Photophobia is a sign of meningeal irritation, but is also associated with several other neurological and ocular disorders.

Photophobia occurs in more than 80% of patients with migraine.[8]

4

Pinpoint pupils

Relevant neuroanatomy and topographical anatomy

Central pathways
- Kappa-1 (κ_1) receptor
- Alpha-2 (α_2) receptor

Sympathetic pathway
FIRST-ORDER NEURON
- Hypothalamus

↓
- Sympathetic fibres, brainstem

↓
- Sympathetic fibres, intermediate horn, spinal cord

↓
SECOND-ORDER NEURON (PREGANGLIONIC FIBRE)
- Sympathetic trunk

↓
- Superior cervical ganglion C2

↓
THIRD-ORDER NEURON (POSTGANGLIONIC FIBRE)
- Superior cervical ganglion C2

↓
- Ciliary body

↓
× Pupillary dilator muscles

Parasympathetic pathway
- Edinger–Westphal nucleus, midbrain

↓
- Oculomotor nerve (CNIII)

↓
- Ciliary ganglion

↓
- Short ciliary nerves

↓
- Neuromuscular junction

↓
× Pupillary constrictor muscle
⇒ Iris

CLINICAL PEARL

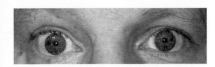

FIGURE 4.1
Bilateral pinpoint pupils, less than 2 mm
in diameter and symmetric

*Murphy SM et al., Conduction block and tonic
pupils in Charcot-Marie-Tooth disease caused
by a myelin protein zero p.Ile112Thr mutation.*
Neuromuscular Disorders 2011; 21(3):
223–226, Copyright © 2010 Elsevier B.V.

Description
Pinpoint pupils are symmetric,
constricted pupils with a diameter
<2 mm.

Condition/s associated with[10-13]

Common
- Opioid – morphine, heroin
- Senile miosis

Less common
- Pontine haemorrhage
- Cholinergic toxicity – organophosphate poisoning
- Upward transtentorial herniation
- Central α-2 agonist – clonidine, dexmedetomidine
- Beta-adrenergic antagonist – carvedilol, timolol

Mechanism/s
The causes of pinpoint pupils are:
- opioid effect
- pontine haemorrhage
- cholinergic toxicity
- α-2 agonist effect
- cerebral herniation with pontine compression
- beta-blocker effect
- senile miosis in normal ageing.

Opioid effect
Binding of opioids at central kappa-1
(κ_1) receptors causes miosis.[10] Not all
opioids cause pupillary constriction
due to heterogenous binding affinity
at κ_1 receptors. Patients taking
meperidine, propoxyphene and
pentazocine may not have pupillary
constriction.[10,11]

Pontine haemorrhage
Pontine haemorrhage disrupts the
descending sympathetic fibres in the
pons, resulting in unopposed
parasympathetic input and bilateral
miosis.[12] Associated features include
profound bilateral cranial nerve signs
(e.g. facial nerve palsy, abducens
nerve palsy), motor long tract signs,
coma and cerebral herniation.

Cholinergic toxicity
Cholinergic toxicity causes bilateral
miosis due to potentiation of
muscarinic receptors at the
neuromuscular junction. Muscarinic
stimulation also results in diarrhoea,
urination, bradycardia,
bronchorrhoea, bronchospasm,
excitation of skeletal muscle,
lacrimation and gastrointestinal
distress.[13] Causes of cholinergic
toxicity include organophosphate and
carbamate toxicity (e.g. insecticide
poisoning).

4

α-2 agonist effect

Clonidine is a central alpha-2 ($α_2$) receptor agonist that inhibits central sympathetic outflow. Inhibition of norepinephrine release causes decreased sympathetic outflow, resulting in bilateral miosis.[14–16]

Cerebral herniation with pontine compression

Central transtentorial herniation, cerebellotonsillar herniation and upward transtentorial herniation cause bilateral miosis due to compression of the pons.[17] Central transtentorial herniation is typically caused by an expanding vertex, frontal lobe or occipital lobe lesion.[17] Cerebellotonsillar herniation is most commonly caused by a cerebellar mass or rapid displacement of the brainstem.[17,18] Upward transtentorial herniation typically results from an expanding posterior fossa lesion.[17]

Beta-blocker effect

Beta-adrenergic antagonism relaxes the pupillary dilator muscle and results in miosis.

Senile miosis in normal ageing

With normal ageing, the pupils decrease in size and have a decreased mydriatic response in low light conditions.[19]

Sign value

Pinpoint pupils are associated with several toxicological and neurological disorders. The most common rapidly reversible cause of coma with pinpoint pupils is opioid toxicity.

Parasympathetic and sympathetic innervation of the iris muscles

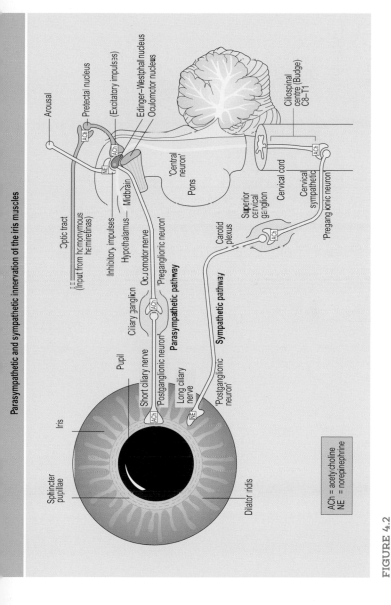

FIGURE 4.2

Parasympathetic and sympathetic pathways innervating the iris muscles

Reproduced, with permission, from Yanoff M, Duker JS, Ophthalmology, 3rd edn, St Louis: Mosby, 2008: Fig 9-19-5.

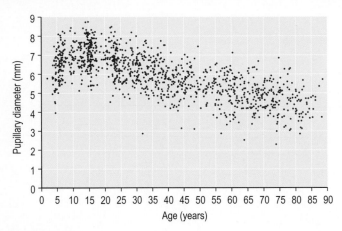

FIGURE 4.3
Changes in pupillary size (horizontal diameter) in darkness at various ages

Reproduced, with permission, from Dyck PJ, Thomas PK, Peripheral Neuropathy, *4th edn, Philadelphia: Saunders, 2005: Fig 9-5.*

References

1. Rucker JC. Cranial neuropathies. In: Bradley WG, Daroff RB, Fenichel G, et al., editors. *Neurology in Clinical Practice*. 5th ed. Philadelphia: Butterworth-Heinemann; 2008.

2. Saliba DL. Reliable block of the gag reflex in one minute or less. *J Clin Anesth* 2009;**21**(6):463.

3. Meeker HG, Magalee R. The conservative management of the gag reflex in full denture patients. *N Y State Dent J* 1986;**52**:11–14.

4. Murphy WM. A clinical survey of gagging patients. *J Prosthet Dent* 1979;**42**:145–8.

5. Wilks CG, Marks IM. Reducing hypersensitive gagging. *Br Dent J* 1983;**155**:263–5.

6. Davies AE. Pharyngeal sensation and gag reflex in healthy subjects. *Lancet* 1995;**345**(8945):487–8.

7. Stringham JM, Fuld K, Wenzel AJ. Spatial properties of photophobia. *Invest Ophthalmol Vis Sci* 2004;**45**:3838–48.

8. Brandt JD. Congenital glaucoma. In: Yanoff M, Duker JS, editors. *Ophthalmology*. 3rd ed. St Louis: Mosby; 2008.

9. Oleson J. Migraine: a neural pathway for photophobia in migraine. *Nat Rev Neurol* 2010;**6**:241–2.

10. Yip L, McGarbane B, Borron SW. Opioids. In: Shannon MW, Borron SW, Burns MJ, editors. *Haddad and Winchester's Clinical Management of Poisoning and Drug Overdose*. 4th ed. Philadelphia: Saunders; 2007.

11. Ghoneum MM, Dhanaraj J, Choi WW. Comparison of four opioid analgesics as supplements to nitrous anesthesia. *Clin Pharmacol Ther* 1984;**63**(4):405–12.

12. Crocco TJ, Tadros A, Kothari RU. Stroke. In: Marx JA, Hockberger RS, Walls RM, et al., editors. *Rosen's Emergency Medicine*. 7th ed. Philadelphia: Mosby; 2010.

13. Meehan TJ, Bryant SM, Aks SE. Drugs of abuse: the highs and lows of altered mental states in the emergency department. *Emerg Med Clin North Am* 2010;**28**:663–82.

14. Reid J. Alpha-adrenergic receptors and blood pressure control. *Am J Cardiol* 1986;**57**:6E–12E.

15. Van Zweiten PA. Overview of alpha-2-adrenoreceptor agonists with central action. *Am J Cardiol* 1986;**57**:3E–5E.

16. Hoffman BB, Lefkowitz RJ. Alpha-adrenergic receptor subtypes. *N Engl J Med* 1980;**302**:1390–6.

17. Biros MH, Heegaard WG. Head injury. In: Marx JA, Hockberger RS, Walls RM, et al., editors. *Rosen's Emergency Medicine*. 7th ed. Philadelphia: Mosby; 2010.

18. Greenberg M. *Handbook of Neurosurgery*. 5th ed. New York: Thieme; 2001.

19. Crouch ER Jr, Crouch ER, Grant T. Ophthalmology. In: Rakel RE, editor. *Textbook of Family Medicine*. 7th ed. Philadelphia: Saunders; 2007.

4

CHAPTER 5

GASTROENTEROLOGICAL SIGNS

Ascites

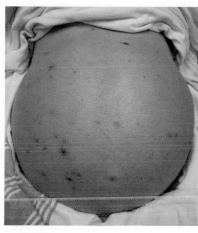

FIGURE 5.1
A person with massive ascites caused by portal hypertension due to cirrhosis
Copyright James Heilman MD.

Although itself not strictly a sign, a variety of clinical signs indicate the presence of ascites. Having an understanding of the different causes of ascites will assist with interpretation of additional signs present on physical examination.

Description

A pathological accumulation of fluid in the peritoneal cavity.

Condition/s associated with

As in oedema, variations in oncotic and hydrostatic pressure and vascular wall integrity are central to the development of ascites (see 'Peripheral oedema' in Chapter 2, 'Cardiovascular signs'). All the pathologies that create ascites effect one or more of these factors.

The causes of ascites can be broadly arranged into four categories according to mechanism (see Table 5.1).

Mechanism/s

Peripheral arterial vasodilatation theory

This hypothesis, shown in Figure 5.2, combines two premises: the 'underfill' and 'overflow' theories. Key initiating elements in both are *portal hypertension* and *nitric oxide-induced splanchnic vasodilatation.*

- *Underfill theory:* Imbalance in hydrostatic versus oncotic pressure causes the intravascular fluid to leak into the peritoneal cavity.[1] The resulting low blood volume activates the renin–angiotensin–aldosterone (RAA) pathway and the sympathetic nervous system to commence renal sodium and fluid retention, in an attempt to maintain volume.[1] As more volume is retained the hydrostatic pressure in the sinusoids causes fluid to be pushed out into the interstitial space. If the patient's lymphatic system is not robust enough to export the additional fluid away,

TABLE 5.1
Causes of ascites

Fluid imbalance (arterial vasodilatation theory)		Exudative
Cirrhosis – common		Exudate-secreting tumours (peritoneal carcinomatosis)
Congestive heart failure – common		Infections (e.g. TB)
Myxoedema		Inflammatory disease (e.g. SLE)
Budd–Chiari syndrome		
Chylous		**Nephrogenic**
Obstruction (e.g. malignant lymphoma)		Haemodialysis
Iatrogenic (e.g. transection of the lymphatics)		Nephrotic syndrome
Retroperitoneal lymph node dissection		

it spills over into the peritoneal cavity to form ascites.

- *Overflow theory:* Primary renal sodium retention in patients with cirrhosis causes intravascular hypervolaemia. This increase in intravascular fluid, in turn, causes increased hydrostatic pressure that forces fluid to overflow into the peritoneal cavity.[2]

Further research following these two theories found that portal hypertension causes the release of nitric oxide and splanchnic bed vasodilatation, which reduces effective arterial blood flow to the kidneys. The RAAS is employed to increase plasma volume, further contributing to fluid overload and ascites.[3–5]

Contrary to popular belief, hypoalbuminaemia and low oncotic pressure have NOT been shown to play a substantial role in the development of ascites.[6]

Liver disease

In liver cirrhosis, destruction of the normal architecture, fibrosis and other structural changes contribute to increased sinusoidal pressure and raised *portal hypertension*. Exacerbating this is the presence of defective nitric oxide synthesis in the liver (responsible for vasodilatation) and the presence of vasoconstrictors, including endothelin,[6] angiotensin II, catecholamines and leukotrienes, all of which serve to favour sinusoidal constriction and the development of portal hypertension,[6] with the resultant driving hydrostatic force pushing fluid out into the peritoneal cavity.

Splanchnic vasodilatation, as mentioned above, is crucial to the

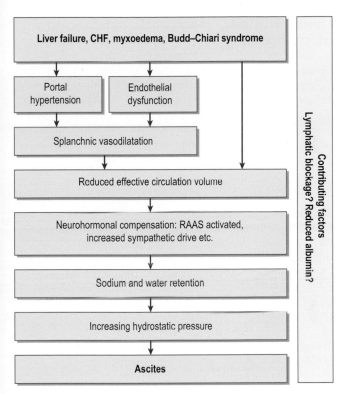

FIGURE 5.2
Mechanisms in the development of ascites

development of ascites. It is thought that vasodilatation of the splanchnic bed is caused by the release of vasodilators, either due to sheer stress in the splanchnic circulation or as a result of neurohormonal signalling from the liver to the brain.[6-8] Nitric oxide, although decreased in the liver, is present and released in increased quantities from the systemic endothelium.[6] Other vasodilators, including calcitonin gene-related peptide (CGRP) and adrenomedulin, have also been implicated.[6]

As a result of this splanchnic vasodilatation, systemic vascular resistance falls, leading to decreased effective blood volume and, ultimately, the activation of the sympathetic and renin–aldosterone systems, and salt and water retention.

Finally, renal dysfunction is also seen in cirrhotic liver patients, with a reduction in GFR and salt and water excretion further contributing to the development of fluid retention and ascites.[6]

Congestive heart failure, Budd–Chiari syndrome

People with these conditions are thought to develop ascites because of reduced effective arterial volumes, leading to activation of the RAAS and salt and fluid retention (underfill theory).[3–5,9,10] Figure 5.3 shows the postulated mechanism of fluid retention and ascites in heart failure.

Nephrotic syndrome

Hypo-albuminaemia is universal in patients with nephrotic syndrome; however, the development of ascites in these patients is not solely caused by low albumin. Though not completely understood, ascites in this setting is likely to be much more complex and low albumin not the predominant mechanism.

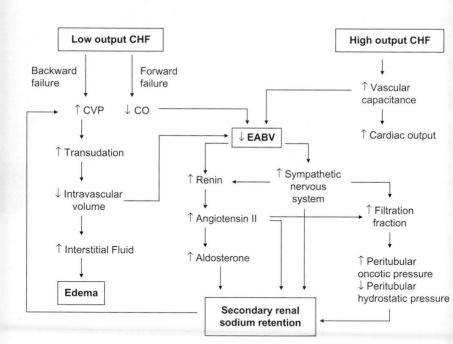

FIGURE 5.3

High-output and low-output cardiac failure

'Summary of the pathways leading to renal sodium retention in low and high-ouput congestive heart failure'. (CO: cardiac output; EABV: effective arterial blood volume; CVP: central venous pressure).

Alpern R, Caplan M, Moe O. Seldin and Giebisch's The Kidney 5th edition (2013). Elsevier.

Intra-renal pathology leading to *inadequate salt excretion* may play a role. Increased tubular reabsorption of salt has been demonstrated in animal models of nephrotic syndrome[3] and may also play a role in human pathology.

'Underfilling' may also play a role in some patients who have proteinuria and hypoalbuminaemia, contributing to a decreased circulating volume and activation of compensatory mechanisms, resulting in salt and water retention.[3]

These mechanisms have been summarised in Figure 5.4.

In a study looking at patients with nephrotic syndrome and ascites, concomitant liver disease and/or a degree of heart failure were also present and contributory to ascitic fluid development,[11] probably via a decrease in effective circulating volume and activation of RAAS and

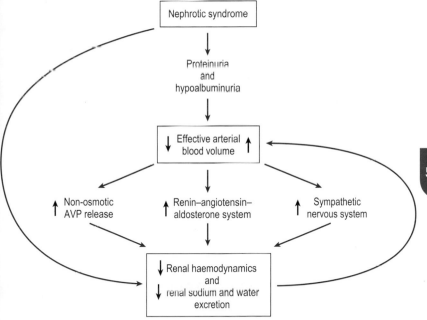

FIGURE 5.4
Nephrotic syndrome
The albuminuria and decrease in plasma oncotic pressure initiate the underfilling in nephrotic syndrome. Renal impairment and intra-renal factors may intervene, however, and in some circumstances restore or even expand effective blood volume. AVP = arginine vasopressin.

Schrier R. Pathogenesis of sodium and water retention in high output and low output cardiac failure, nephrotic syndrome, cirrhosis and pregnancy. First of 2 parts. NEJM 1988; 319(16): Fig 3. Reprinted with permission from Massachusetts Medical Society.

the sympathetic nervous system, with resulting salt and fluid retention.

Myxoedema mechanism/s

The mechanism of ascites in hypothyroidism or myxoedema is unclear. Previously two theories have existed. Firstly, that low levels of thyroid hormones cause *increased extravasation* of *plasma proteins* due to increased capillary permeability combined with a lack of compensatory lymphatic and protein flow return rate to the plasma.[12,13]

The second theory suggested that *hyaluronic acid* accumulates in the skin and produces oedema through its ability to absorb or adsorp water (i.e. its ability to attract and hold water molecules), although there is minimal evidence for this direct effect.[12,14] The hyaluronic acid is also thought to form complexes with albumin which prevents it from being picked up and returned to the circulation via the lymphatic system.[12]

In severe hypothyroidism, a variety of changes occur in the cardiovascular system and renal system including decreased myocardial contractility and renal dysfunction with inability to excrete excess water (free water clearance), which may also contribute to fluid retention. Direct research on these changes and ascites is lacking.

Exudative ascites

Exudative ascites may be caused by:

- increased intraperitoneal oncotic pressure (e.g. peritoneal carcinomatosis causes the tumour cells lining the peritoneum to produce exudates)
- disruption of vessel wall integrity that allows fluid to leak through (e.g. patients with systemic lupus erythematosus can develop an inflammatory serositis, leading to exudate).[10,15]

Chylous ascites

Obstruction of lymphatic flow is the main underlying mechanism. This can be due to a pathological obstruction raising lymphatic pressures, resulting in fluid being pushed out and/or disrupting vessel integrity leading to leakage. Examples of these two scenarios are malignant lymphoma and surgical rupture of lymph nodes or vessels.[16,17]

Nephrogenic – haemodialysis

The causes of ascites in patients who receive haemodialysis are largely unknown. One possible explanation is that uraemia induces an inflammatory response that causes immune-complex formation and obstruction of lymphatic channels.[18,19]

Ascites clinical signs

Several clinical signs indicate the presence of ascites but none indicate the underlying cause.

Sign value

The presence of ascites in a patient with liver disease suggests the presence of underlying cirrhosis with a PLR of 7.2 (CI 2.9-12),[20] and thus is helpful in understanding the extent and chronicity of disease.

Appreciating the mechanism behind ascites, and in particular cirrhosis-induced ascites, has substantial value in aiding understanding of the disease state and its sequelae, as well as insight into how therapeutic interventions act. In Figure 5.5, the pathogenesis of ascites is shown along with targets for various treatment opportunities.

In terms of the various signs that are used to detect the presence of ascites, there are variable sensitivities and specificities. In patients with abdominal distension, the sign with the best positive likelihood ratio (most likely to have ascites) is the fluid wave.[21] The best signs to exclude ascites are the absence of oedema (NLR 0.2) and absence of flank dullness.[21]

Serum albumin/ascitic gradient (SAAG) – a guide to pathophysiology and diagnosis of the sign

The serum albumin ascitic gradient (SAAG) is used to identify the presence of portal hypertension.

SAAG = serum albumin – ascitic fluid albumin

The theory is based on Starling's forces between the serum and ascitic fluid and the relationship between oncotic pressure, hydrostatic pressure and endothelial permeability.

In conditions when hydrostatic pressure is elevated (e.g. in portal hypertension), fluid is pushed out into the abdomen, and thus the serum albumin level becomes more concentrated compared to the ascitic fluid albumin, and the gap or gradient widens.

Conditions in which there is either low albumin in the serum (e.g. nephrotic syndrome) or protein leakage into the peritoneal cavity (e.g. inflammation, malignancy) result in higher protein and/or albumin content entering the peritoneal cavity, creating a low SAAG. Table 5.2 shows examples of causes of both high and low albumin gradients.

5

Ascites

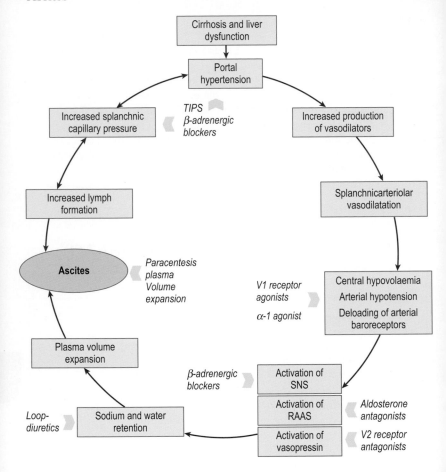

FIGURE 5.5
Pathophysiology of the development of ascites in cirrhosis and potential targets for treatment
SNS = sympathetic nervous system; RAAS = renin–angiotensin–aldosterone system; AVP = arginine vasopressin; TIPS = transjugular intrahepatic portosystemic shunt.

Moller S, Henriksen J, Bendtsen F. Ascites: pathogenesis and therapeutic principles. Scandinavian Journal of Gastroenterology *2009; 44: 902–911, Fig 1, Informa PLC.*

TABLE 5.2

Serum albumin ascitic gradient and pathologies

High albumin gradient (SAAG >11.1g/l)	Low albumin gradient (SAAG <11.1g/l)
Cirrhosis	Peritoneal carcinomatosis
Alcoholic hepatitis	Pancreatitis
Heart failure	Nephrotic syndrome
Budd–Chiari syndrome	Bacterial peritonitis
Portal vein thrombosis	

5

Bowel sounds: absent

Description

As the name implies, the complete absence of bowel sounds on auscultation. How long one must listen before bowel sounds may be called absent is not clear, with times quoted anywhere from 1–5 minutes.

Condition/s associated with

More common

- Intestinal obstruction
- Paralytic ileus of any cause, e.g.:
  » Infection
  » Trauma
  » Bowel obstruction
  » Hypokalaemia
  » Vascular ischaemia
  » Side effect to drugs

Less common

- Mesenteric ischaemia
- Pseudo-obstruction (Ogilvie syndrome)

General mechanism/s

Absent bowel sounds may be caused by obstruction of an active intestine, resulting in an inability to push food or fluid through, or by an inactive bowel that is not undergoing peristalsis.

Bowel obstruction

In a mechanical obstruction due to any cause (hernia, volvulus, adhesion), the intestines are pushing against a fixed object. The normal oscillatory movement of food and water is not happening (as in a blocked pipe), so no sound is produced. If the obstruction continues, inflammation occurs and, if vascular supply is compromised, normal peristalsis may also stop.

Infection

Although not entirely explained, there is evidence that the lipopolysaccharides (LPS) present on Gram-negative bacteria initiate an inflammatory response in the intestinal smooth muscle layer, which then reduces smooth muscle contractility, causing an ileus.[22]

Postoperative ileus

It is hypothesised that manipulation of the small intestine leads to postoperative ileus by promoting *inflammation of the smooth muscle layer*, which then causes a reduction in intestinal smooth muscle activity.[23]

There is also evidence to suggest that bacterial overgrowth occurs within the gut postoperatively and that the increased presence of bacteria and lipopolysaccharides contributes to inflammation caused by manipulation.[24]

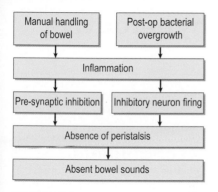

FIGURE 5.6
Possible postoperative ileus mechanism

The means by which inflammation causes ileus is likely to be related to the suppression of synaptic circuits of the enteric plexus, which organise normal propulsion of the intestines.[25] This suppression is caused by pre-synaptic inhibition of enteric motor neurons and/or continuous discharge of inhibitory neurons.

Hypokalaemia

Potassium is needed for normal polarisation and repolarisation of muscle cells. Hypokalaemia causes a *hyperpolarisation* of muscle cells, reducing excitability of the neurons and therefore smooth muscle activity; leading to ileus.

Pseudo-obstruction

The cause or mechanism of pseudo-obstruction, also known as Ogilvie syndrome, is not clear.

It is thought that an imbalance of autonomic innervation causes a functional bowel obstruction. Normal sacral parasympathetic tone is disrupted, causing an adynamic distal colon. Other studies suggest increased sympathetic tone is the cause – leading to decreased gut motility and sphincter closing. Peristalsis may be absent or impaired.

5

Bowel sounds: hyperactive (borborygmus)

Description

Frequent, loud, gurgling or 'rushing' bowel sounds that sometimes may be clearly heard even without a stethoscope.

Condition/s associated with:

More common

- Bowel obstruction
- Crohn's disease/ulcerative colitis
- Food hypersensitivity
- Gastroenteritis
- Normal

Less common

- Gastrointestinal haemorrhage

Mechanism/s

When obstruction is present, the bowel increases peristalsis in an attempt to overcome the blockage.

Coffee ground vomiting/ bloody vomitus/ haematemesis

Description

The vomiting of red blood or a coffee-ground-like substance. Haematemesis refers to the coughing up or vomiting of frank red blood.

Condition/s associated with

- Upper gastrointestinal bleeding[26]

More common

- Peptic ulcer disease
- Gastritis
- Oesophagitis
- Oesophageal varices

Less common

- Mallory–Weiss tear
- Vascular
- Tumour
- Vasculitis

General mechanism/s

Tearing or rupture of a blood vessel within the gastrointestinal tract, regardless of cause or aetiology, can precipitate haematemesis and/or coffee ground vomitus.

Coffee ground vomits owe their distinctive appearance to blood that has been oxidised by gastric acid, similar to malaena. It therefore indicates that the blood and/or bleeding has been present for some time, and potentially is higher up in the gastrointestinal tract (i.e. the duodenum or stomach).

Peptic ulcer disease

Inflammation and erosion of the normal mucosal surface into an underlying artery causes bleeding. Blood irritates the gut and is vomited back up.

Mallory–Weiss tear

Bleeding is due to longitudinal mucosal lacerations at the gastro-oesophageal junction or gastric cardia.

The mechanism behind Mallory–Weiss tears is not completely known but the theory is summarised in Figure 5.7. The sudden rise in abdominal/intragastric pressure from vomiting causes an increase in pressure across the gastro-oesophageal junction. This junction is relatively non-compliant and does not distend well with pressure. When the pressure gets high enough or is repeated (with multiple vomits), a mucosal laceration occurs, resulting in bleeding.

5

CLINICAL PEARL

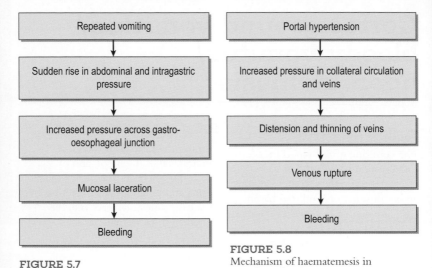

FIGURE 5.7
Mechanism of Mallory–Weiss tear

FIGURE 5.8
Mechanism of haematemesis in oesophageal varices

Oesophageal varices

In any cause of portal hypertension, the rise in portal vein pressure means blood is directed *away* into lower-pressure systems – collateral systems that include the oesophageal veins, abdominal veins and rectal veins. These veins become distended, thinner and more fragile. Rupturing of the thin-walled collateral veins/ varices in the oesophagus causes pooling of blood and haematemesis. Gastric varices may also bleed in patients with portal hypertension.

Sign value

There are a number of causes of upper gastrointestinal bleeding, and other sources of blood coming from the mouth need to be considered (e.g. nose, teeth, sinuses). However, both haematemesis and melaena are valuable signs and warrant immediate investigation, given the potential for catastrophic bleeding.

Guarding

Description

May be voluntary or involuntary in nature.

Voluntary guarding is the conscious contraction of the abdominal musculature, usually in response to fear of pain or anxiety.

Involuntary guarding is discussed under 'Rigidity and involuntary guarding' in this chapter.

Condition/s associated with

Any cause of peritonism:

- Inflammation of any visceral organ
- Abdominal infection
- Bleeding

Mechanism/s

In anticipation of pain the patient contracts the abdominal muscles as a protective response.

Sign value

Despite several studies, the sensitivity and specificity for guarding in the diagnosis of peritonitis is highly variable, ranging from 13–90% for sensitivity and 40–97% for specificity, with a PLR of 2.2 and NLR of 0.6.[21] While imaging modalities are often superior to physical examination in diagnosing specific disorders, the detection of guarding may help the clinician to consider appropriate tests.

5

Haematuria

Description

The presence of red blood cells in the urine. It may be microscopic (i.e. only detected on urinalysis and/or microscopy) or be visible to the naked eye (i.e. macroscopic).

Condition/s associated with

Common

- Kidney stones
- Malignancy
- Trauma to the urinary tract (e.g. infection or instrumentation)

Less common

- Glomerulonephritis – nephritis syndrome
- IgA nephropathy
- Goodpasture's syndrome
- Vasculitis
- Interstitial nephritis
- Polycystic kidneys
- Papillary infarction

Mechanism/s

Bleeding from anywhere in the renal tract will result in haematuria. Figure 5.9 provides an overview of this.

Detailed pathophysiology of each cause of haematuria is outside the scope of this text. In short, disruption of the renal tract, either by an obstruction (stone), altered kidney structure (polycystic kidneys) or immunological deposition may cause destruction of architecture and bring blood into the urinary tract.

Sign value

While transient haematuria (particularly microscopic) is not uncommon and may be benign, persistent haematuria or haematuria with altered renal function and/or other concerning features requires immediate investigation. Painless macroscopic haematuria in an elderly person should be considered a malignancy until proven otherwise.

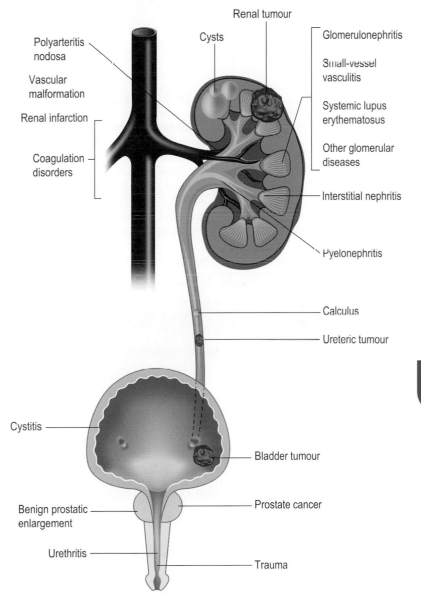

FIGURE 5.9
Causes of haematuria

Walker B, Davidson's Principles and Practice of Medicine, *22nd edn, London: Elsevier 2014: Fig 7.7.*

Jaundice

Description

Yellowing of the skin, sclera and mucous membranes.

Condition/s associated with

There are many different causes of jaundice; they can be grouped as shown in Table 5.3.

Mechanism/s

Jaundice is caused by a build-up of *excess bilirubin which is deposited in the skin and mucous membranes*. Jaundice is not clinically evident until serum bilirubin exceeds 3 mg/L. Defects along the bilirubin pathway (shown in Figure 5.10) lead to increased bilirubin and jaundice.

TABLE 5.3
Causes of jaundice

Pre-hepatic causes	Hepatic causes	Post-hepatic causes
See Chapter 3, 'Haematological and oncological signs'	More common	
	Alcohol	
	Malignancy	
	Viral hepatitis	
	Cirrhosis of the liver	Gallstones
	Cholestasis	
	Drug-induced (e.g. paracetamol)	
	Less common	
	Primary biliary cirrhosis	Pancreatic cancer
	Primary sclerosing cholangitis	Biliary atresia
	Gilbert's syndrome	Cholangiosarcoma
	Crigler–Najjar syndrome	
	Autoimmune hepatitis	

Pre-hepatic

Jaundice in this scenario is due to excessive breakdown of red blood cells and the release of unconjugated bilirubin. See 'Haemolytic/pre-hepatic jaundice' in Chapter 3, 'Haematological and oncological signs'.

Intrahepatic

In this case the liver's *ability to take up bilirubin, bind, conjugate and/or secrete it* into the bile canaliculi is impaired. This can be due to either acquired damage to or necrosis of liver cells or genetic deficiencies in the bilirubin pathway.

Gilbert's syndrome is an example of a genetic deficiency in the bilirubin pathway. A genetic abnormality of the enzyme glucuronyltransferase reduces the liver's ability to conjugate bilirubin. As a result, unconjugated bilirubin cannot be excreted properly and hyperbilirubinaemia occurs to a level that eventually causes jaundice.

Similarly, in Dubin–Johnson syndrome, a genetic defect in a transporter (cMOAT) stops conjugated bilirubin from being secreted effectively, and bilirubin rises, resulting in jaundice.

There are many hepatic causes of jaundice. Any condition that can cause enough damage or destruction to the liver to prevent normal bilirubin processing can cause jaundice. More and less common causes are listed in Table 5.3.

Drug-induced liver injury

A huge number of drugs can cause liver injury and result in jaundice, among other things. A variety of mechanisms have been proposed and include:[27]

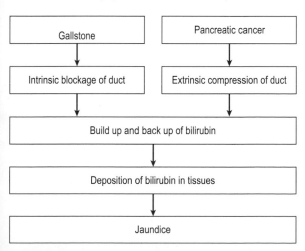

FIGURE 5.10
Example mechanism of post-hepatic jaundice

TABLE 5.4
Mechanisms of common drug-induced liver injury

Drug	Mechanism/s
Augmentin (amoxicillin + clavulanic acid)	Stimulates an immune-driven response, especially in patients with genetic predisposition including: Class I & II HLA DQB1*0602, HLA DRB1*15014
Valproate	Mitochondrial injury Histone deacetylase inhibition
Cyclosporin	Bile salt pump inhibition
Flucloxacillin	Bile salt pump inhibition Immunological hypersensitivity reaction associated with patients with HLA B*5701
Paracetamol	Toxic doses saturate normal metabolism, more substrate is shunted down CYP2E1 metabolism resulting in excess NAPQI, glutathione is depleted and cannot neutralise NAPQI which is toxic to liver cell membranes

- formation of reactive metabolites
- bile salt export pump (BSEP) inhibition – leading to a build-up of bile salts in hepatocytes
- drug transporter/metabolising enzymes modulation
- mitochondrial toxicity[28]
- oxidative stress
- modulating adaptive/innate immune reactions
- biliary epithelial injury
- histone acetylation.

A small selection of pharmaceuticals that can cause jaundice via these pathways is shown in Table 5.4.

FIGURE 5.11
Bilirubin metabolism and elimination

1 Normal bilirubin production from haem (0.2–0.3 g/day) is derived primarily from the breakdown of senescent circulating erythrocytes.
2 Extrahepatic bilirubin is bound to serum albumin and delivered to the liver.
3 Hepatocellular uptake and 4 glucuronidation in the endoplasmic reticulum generate bilirubin, which is water-soluble and readily excreted into bile.
5 Gut bacteria deconjugate the bilirubin and degrade it to colourless urobilinogens. The urobilinogens and the residue of intact pigments are excreted in the faeces, with some reabsorption and excretion into urine.

Reproduced, with permission, from Kumar V, Abbas AK, Fausto N, Aster JC, Robbins and Cotran Pathologic Basis of Disease, Professional Edition, 8th edn, Philadelphia: Saunders, 2009: Fig 18-4.

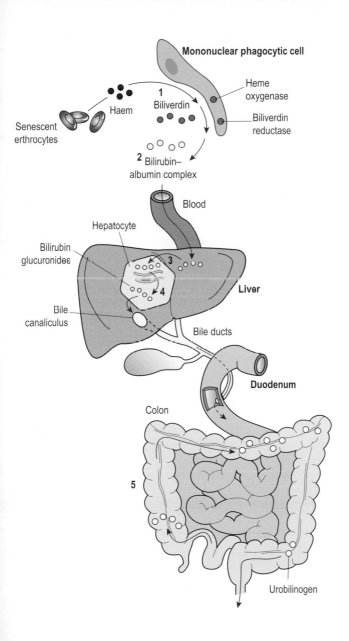

Dark-coloured urine/pale-coloured stools of biliary obstruction

Often associated with post-hepatic or obstructive jaundice is the sign of 'dark urine/pale stools'. In healthy people, unconjugated bilirubin is bound tightly to albumin and cannot be excreted in the urine (it cannot 'fit' through the glomerulus of the kidney). However, in patients with obstructive jaundice, conjugated bilirubin binds less tightly to albumin and may be excreted in the urine, giving it a dark tea colour.

Bile duct obstruction does not allow excretion of bilirubin into the intestines; therefore, the stool does not accumulate the bile pigments that normally make it dark in colour, and the patient will have a noticeably pale bowel motion.

Post-hepatic

Post-hepatic jaundice is caused by a *blockage of bile ducts* preventing the excretion of conjugated bilirubin. Bilirubin backs up through the liver into the bloodstream.

Sign value

Jaundice is an important clinical sign and must be identified and investigated. If found, the clinician should attempt to identify other presenting features which may point to the cause of jaundice (e.g. signs of chronic liver disease: palmar erythema, spider naevi, ascites, a palpable gallbladder, lymphadenopathy). In almost 80% of cases one can identify a hepatic versus post-hepatic cause of jaundice at the bedside, resulting in appropriate test ordering and a much shorter differential diagnosis list.[29]

Melaena

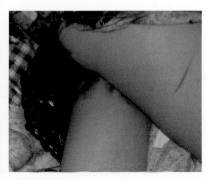

FIGURE 5.12
Melaena

Malik A et al. Dengue hemorrhagic fever outbreak in children in Port Sudan. Journal of Infection and Public Health *2010; 4(1): Fig 6.*

Description
Black, tarry, foul-smelling stools.

Condition/s associated with
- Gastrointestinal haemorrhage/ bleed

More common
- Peptic ulcer disease
- Oesophageal varices
- Oesophagitis
- Gastritis

Less common
- Mallory–Weiss tear
- Neoplasm

Mechanism/s
Bleeding from any cause in the upper gastrointestinal tract can result in melaena. It is often said that bleeding must begin above the ligament of Treitz; however, this is not always the case. The black, foul-smelling nature of the stool is due to the *oxidation of iron from the haemoglobin*, as it passes through the gastrointestinal tract.

Sign value
If present, melaena requires complete investigation, bearing in mind that it is not necessarily specific to the location of the bleed.

5

Oliguria/anuria

Description

Although not easily observed as a sign, urine output can be enquired about and a routine fluid balance check is included in the review of many conditions. Oliguria is described as less than 400 mL urine output per day in adults and less than 0.5 mL/kg/hr in children. Anuria refers to urine output of less than 100 mL per day in adults.

Condition/s associated with

Like the classifications of acute renal failure, the conditions associated with oliguria can be split into 'Pre-renal', 'Renal' and 'Post-renal'.

Mechanisms/s

The aetiology of every condition that can result in low urine output is out of the scope of this text; however, brief mechanisms for groups of conditions are provided below.

Pre-renal

Oliguria resulting from pre-renal causes is principally due to *reduced renal perfusion*. Adequate perfusion of the kidneys is reliant on fluid (blood), adequate pipes (veins and arteries) and an adequate pump (heart). Problems with one or more of these three elements (e.g. dehydration [lack of fluid], sepsis [leaky pipes], heart failure [pump]) results in under-perfusion of the kidneys. The kidneys are exquisitely sensitive to decreased circulating volume or flow and have a number of compensatory mechanisms to activate (e.g. the renin–angiotensin II system), which ultimately results in retention of salt and water, and therefore less urine being passed.

TABLE 5.5
Classifications of oliguria

Pre-renal	Renal	Post-renal
Dehydration	Acute tubular necrosis	Bladder outlet obstruction (e.g. stones/tumours)
Blood loss	Drugs	Bilateral ureteric obstruction
Sepsis	Toxins	
Cardiac failure	Glomerulonephritis	
Burns	Vascular (e.g. renal artery thrombosis)	
Drugs	Interstitial nephritis	
Anaphylaxis		

CLINICAL PEARL

Renal

Intrinsic renal impairment causing oliguria results from structural damage to the kidneys. If there is significant enough insult to the renal architecture, the kidneys cannot filter or function to produce urine.

Post-renal

Obstruction of the ureters, bladder or urethra will prevent urine from being passed. If this occurs for long enough it can cause intrinsic damage to the kidneys, further affecting urine production.

Sign value

Oliguria is an essential sign to be aware of and can help guide therapy and also alert the clinician to developing pathology.

5

References

1. Sherlock S, Shaldon S. The aetiology and management of ascites in patients with hepatic cirrhosis: a review. *Gut* 1963;**4**:95–105.

2. Lieberman FL, Denison EK, Reynolds TB. The relationship of plasma volume, portal hypertension, ascites, and renal sodium retention in cirrhosis: the overflow theory of ascites formation. *Ann NY Acad Sci* 1970;**70**:202–12.

3. Schrier RW. Pathogenesis of sodium and water retention in high-output and low-output cardiac failure, nephrotic syndrome, cirrhosis, and pregnancy: first of two parts. *N Engl J Med* 1988;**319**:1065–72.

4. Schrier RW. Pathogenesis of sodium and water retention in high-output and low-output cardiac failure, nephrotic syndrome, cirrhosis, and pregnancy: second of two parts. *N Engl J Med* 1988;**319**:1127–32.

5. Chiprut RO, Knudsen KB, Liebermann TR, et al. Myxedema ascites. *Am J Digest Dis* 1976;**21**:807–8.

6. Moller S, Henriksen J, Bendtsen F. Ascites: pathogenesis and therapeutic principles. *Scand J Gastroenterol* 2009;**44**:902–11.

7. Moller S, Henriksen JH. The systemic circulation in cirrhosis. In: Gines P, Arroyo V, Rodes J, Schrier RW, editors. *Ascites and renal dysfunction in liver disease*. Malden: Blackwell; 2005. pp. 139–55.

8. Wiest R. Splanchnic and systemic vasodilatation: the experimental models. *J Clinc Gastroenterol* 2007;**41**:S272–87.

9. De Castro F, Bonacini M, Walden JM, et al. Myxedema ascites: report of two cases and review of the literature. *J Clin Gastroenterol* 1991;**13**:411–14.

10. Yu AS, Hu KQ. Management of ascites. *Clin Liver Dis* 2001;**5**(2):541–68.

11. Ackerman Z. Ascites in nephrotic syndrome: incidence, patients' characteristics and complications. *J Clin Gastroenterol* 1996;**22**(1):31–4.

12. Jeong-Seon J, et al. Myxedema ascites: case report and literature review. *J Korean Med Sci* 2006;**21**:761–4.

13. Parving H-H, et al. Mechanisms of edema formation in myxedema increased protein extravasation and relatively slow lymphatic drainage. *NEJM* 1979;**301**:460–5.

14. Bonvalet JP. Myxedema with inappropriate antiduresis and hyperaldosteronism. *Ann Med Interne* 1970;**121**:949–55.

15. Pockros PJ, Esrason KT, Nguyen C, et al. Mobilization of malignant ascites with diuretics is dependent on ascitic fluid characteristics. *Gastroenterology* 1992;**103**:1302–6.

16. Brown MW, Burk RF. Development of intractable ascites following upper abdominal surgery in patients with cirrhosis. *Am J Med* 1986;**80**:879–83.

17. Miedema EB, Bissada NK, Finkbeiner AE, et al. Chylous ascites complicating retroperitoneal lymphadenectomy for testis tumors: management with peritoneovenous shunting. *J Urol* 1978;**120**:377–82.

18. Bichler T, Dudley DA. Nephrogenous ascites. *Am J Gastroenterol* 1983;**77**:73–4.

19. Han SHB, Reynolds TB, Fong TL. Nephrogenic ascites: analysis of 16 cases and review of the literature. *Medicine* 1998;**77**:233–45.

20. Udell JA, et al. Does this patient with liver disease have cirrhosis? *JAMA* 2012;**307**(8):832–42.

21. McGee S. *Evidence Based Physical Diagnosis*. 3rd ed. St Louis: Elsevier; 2012.

22. Eskandari MK, Kalff JC, Billiar TR, et al. Lipopolysaccharide activates the muscularis macrophage network and suppresses circular smooth muscle activity. *Am J Physiol* 1997;**273**:G727–34.

23. Kalff JC, Schraut WH, Simmons RL, Bauer AJ. Surgical manipulation of the gut elicits an intestinal muscularis inflammatory response resulting in paralytic ileus. *Ann Surg* 1998;**228**:625–53.

24. Schwarz NT, Simmons RL, Bauer AJ. Minor intraabdominal injury followed by low dose LPS administration act synergistically to induce ileus. *Neurogastroenterol Motil* 2000;**11**(2):288.

25. Wood J. Chapter 26: Neurogastroenterology and gastrointestinal motility. In: Rhoades RA, Tanner GA, editors. *Medical Physiology*. 2nd ed. Philadelphia: Lippincott Williams & Wilkins; 2003.

26. Palmer K. Management of haematemesis and melaena. *Postgrad Med J* 2004;**80**: 399–404.

27. Yuan L. Mechanisms of drug induced liver injury. *Clin Liver Dis* 2013;**17**(4):507–18.

28. Aleo MD, et al. Human drug-induced liver injury severity is highly associated with dual inhibition of liver mitochondrial function and bile salt export pump. *Hepatology* 2014;**60**(3):1015–22.

29. O'Connor KW, Snodgrass PJ, Swonder JE, et al. A blinded prospective study comparing four current noninvasive approaches in the differential diagnosis of medical versus surgical jaundice. *Gastroenterology* 1983;**84**(6):1498–504.

5

CHAPTER 6

ENDOCRINOLOGICAL SIGNS

Bruising

Description

This refers to bruising caused by minimal trauma (i.e. an insult that would not normally result in a bruise).

Condition/s associated with

- Cushing's syndrome
- Renal failure with uraemia

See 'Ecchymoses, purpura and petechiae' in Chapter 3, 'Haematological and oncological signs', for further causes.

Mechanism/s

Cushing's syndrome

Loss of subcutaneous connective tissue, due to the catabolic effects of glucocorticoids, exposes underlying vessels prone to rupture. It is a similar mechanism to that of striae.

Renal failure with uraemia

The mechanism is complex and unclear.

It is thought that uraemic blood alters *platelet function, causing ineffective activation, aggregation and attachment* to blood vessel endothelium[1] rather than thrombocytopenia.

The major elements involved in this clotting dysfunction are shown in Figure 6.1.

- *Platelet function.* Defects in secretion of pro-aggregation factors, an imbalance between platelet agonists and inhibitors, excess parathyroid hormone (which inhibits platelet aggregation) and decreased thromboxane A2 all contribute to either ineffective activation or aggregation.[1]

- *Vessel wall attachment.* Normally, platelets have certain proteins that are responsible for attachment to both other platelets and vessel endothelium – helping clot formation and stopping bleeding. Uraemic toxins cause drops in glycoprotein[2,3] GP 1b and dysfunction in other receptors (α_{IIb} β_3) that are necessary for platelet attachment to blood vessel walls, as well as normal interaction with vWF and fibrinogen, thus inhibiting effective platelet clotting as well as attachment. Rises in other inhibitors, such as NO and PGI$_2$, are also present in uraemic patients, contributing to defective platelet clotting and thus easy bruising.[1]

- *Anaemia.* Red blood cells are integral to normal platelet activation and the clotting process. In ordinary quantities, they 'push' platelets towards the

6

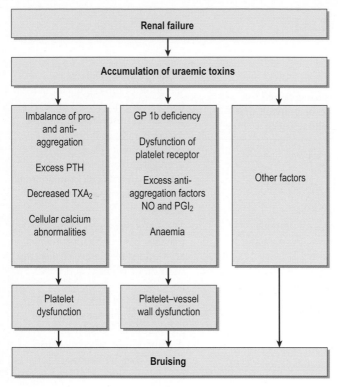

FIGURE 6.1
Mechanism of bruising in renal failure

vascular endothelium and increase ADP-enhancing platelet activation. Uraemic patients are often anaemic and these regular processes are often diminished or absent, leading to prolonged bleeding time. Some studies have suggested that anaemia is the primary reason for prolonged bleeding time in uraemic patients.[4]

• *Other factors.* Drugs, including cephalosporins and aspirin, have been shown to affect platelet function.

Hypotension

Description
Abnormally low blood pressure, usually less than 100 mmHg systolic.

Condition/s associated with
- Addison's disease
- Hypothyroidism

Mechanism/s
Numerous causes, see Chapter 2, 'Cardiovascular signs'.

Addison's disease
Dehydration and volume loss is the primary cause of hypotension in Addison's disease.

Mineralocorticoids regulate sodium retention and potassium excretion in the urine, sweat, saliva and GI tract. A deficiency of mineralocorticoids and, to a much lesser extent, corticosteroids leads to *salt wasting* and *failure to concentrate urine*, thus producing *decreased circulatory volume, dehydration* and *hypotension*.

Deficiency of glucocorticoids (adrenaline) may also lower the basal tone of the vasculature and, therefore, resting systolic blood pressure.

Hypothyroidism
Thyroid hormones have multiple effects on the cardiovascular system (see 'Thyroid hormone and the cardiovascular system' box and Figure 6.2).

Sign value
A common sign in acute primary adrenal insufficiency – up to 88% of patients exhibit hypotension.[5] However, given the myriad causes of hypotension, its value as an isolated sign is limited. Conversely, the presence of *hyper*tension is a strong negative predictor of a diagnosis of Addison's disease.[6,7]

6

Thyroid hormone and the cardiovascular system

Thyroid hormones have myriad effects on different peripheral tissues and systems. The cardiovascular system is no different and understanding the role of thyroid hormones (in particular T3) will help the clinician identify and interpret signs related to either excess or deficit.

T3 enters the myocyte and binds to nuclear receptors, which then attach to thyroid response elements in target genes. These in turn bind to DNA and regulate gene expression, which has a variety of effects including:[8]

- altered myosin heavy chain expression
- expression of myofibrillin proteins that make up thick filaments
- increased Ca^{2+} ATPase (required for myocardial contraction and relaxation)
- increased beta-adrenergic receptor expression
- altered ion transporter expression.

T3 also has direct effects on peripheral vascular resistance, lowering it when present in excess and vice versa.[8] Increased tissue thermogenesis also contributes to decreased peripheral resistance.

Further, T3 can increase EPO, circulating blood volume and preload.

In summary
- increased heart rate, contractility and blood pressure in hyperthyroidism
- in general, the opposite in hypothyroidism

FIGURE 6.2
Mechanisms of action of thyroid hormones and the cardiovascular system
Adapted from Klein I, Ojamaa K. Thyroid hormone and the cardiovascular system. New England Journal of Medicine *2001; 344(7): 501–509, Tables 1 and 2.*

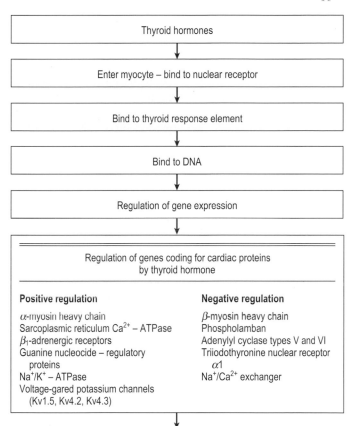

```
┌─────────────────────────────────────────────────────────────┐
│                      Thyroid hormones                         │
└─────────────────────────────────────────────────────────────┘
                              ↓
┌─────────────────────────────────────────────────────────────┐
│          Enter myocyte – bind to nuclear receptor             │
└─────────────────────────────────────────────────────────────┘
                              ↓
┌─────────────────────────────────────────────────────────────┐
│             Bind to thyroid response element                  │
└─────────────────────────────────────────────────────────────┘
                              ↓
┌─────────────────────────────────────────────────────────────┐
│                        Bind to DNA                            │
└─────────────────────────────────────────────────────────────┘
                              ↓
┌─────────────────────────────────────────────────────────────┐
│                Regulation of gene expression                  │
└─────────────────────────────────────────────────────────────┘
                              ↓
```

Regulation of genes coding for cardiac proteins by thyroid hormone

Positive regulation	Negative regulation
α-myosin heavy chain	β-myosin heavy chain
Sarcoplasmic reticulum Ca^{2+} – ATPase	Phospholamban
β_1-adrenergic receptors	Adenylyl cyclase types V and VI
Guanine nucleocide – regulatory proteins	Triiodothyronine nuclear receptor $\alpha 1$
Na^+/K^+ – ATPase	Na^+/Ca^{2+} exchanger
Voltage-gared potassium channels (Kv1.5, Kv4.2, Kv4.3)	

Changes in cardiovascular function associated with thyroid disease

Measure	Normal Range	Values in hyper-thyroidism	Values in hypo-thyroidism
Systemic vascular resistance ($dyn \cdot sec \cdot cm^{-4}$)	1700	700–1200	2100–2700
Heart rate (beats/min)	72–84	88–130	60–80
Ejection fraction (%)	50–60	>60	≤60
Cardiac output (hours/min)	4.0–6.0	>7.0	<4.5
Isovolumic relaxation time (msec)	60–80	25–40	>80
Blood volume (% of normal value)	100	105.5	84.5

Polydipsia

Description

Although strictly more a symptom than a sign, excessive drinking can be witnessed and is often linked to polyuria. Polydipsia is the chronic and excessive sensation of thirst and intake of fluid.[9] Differentiation should be made between true thirst due to dehydration-causing polyuria and that due to a dry mouth alone (due to effects of medicines or local factors).

Condition/s associated with

More common

- Diabetes mellitus
- Diabetes insipidus
- Anticholinergics

Less common

- Hypercalcaemia
- Psychogenic polydipsia
- Sjögren's syndrome
- Primary hyperaldosteronism

Mechanism/s

Often secondary to polyuria and as a response to dehydration (from diabetes mellitus, diabetes insipidus, hypercalcaemia). See 'Polyuria' in this chapter.

Sjögren's syndrome

In Sjögren's syndrome, an autoimmune disorder stops the production of saliva (and affects lacrimal glands). The result of this is a dry mouth, and the patient continues to drink in order to alleviate the discomfort.

Psychogenic polydipsia

This is thought to be a multi-factorial malfunction of the hypothalamic thirst centre, involving the chronic intake of excessive amounts of water, which reset the thirst and ADH cue points. In other words, patients need to drink more to satisfy their feeling of thirst and/or ADH is inappropriately suppressed.

Positive symptoms of schizophrenia, compulsive behaviour, stress reactions, drinking to counteract anticholinergic side effects to drugs and elevated dopamine responses stimulating the thirst centre have all been suggested as possible triggers.

Primary hyperaldosteronism

Excess aldosterone leads to hypokalaemia which, in turn, causes a decrease in aquaporin water tubules in the cortical collecting ducts of the kidneys. With less water able to be reabsorbed, more is excreted, leading to polyuria.

Polyuria

Description

Passing of a large volume of urine within a defined period of time.[9] Although not truly a sign, it is important in a number of endocrinological and renal conditions, and in some settings can be measured.

Condition/s associated with

More common

- Diabetes mellitus
- Diabetes insipidus
- Excess IV fluids
- Osmotic mannitol infusion, radiocontrast media, high-protein tube feeds
- Drugs (e.g. diuretics, lithium)
- Caffeine
- Post-obstructive diuresis

Less common

- Hypokalaemia
- Hypercalcaemia
- Psychogenic polydipsia (e.g. schizophrenia)
- Excess IV fluids
- Cushing's syndrome
- Primary hyperaldosteronism
- Inability to concentrate urine: sickle cell trait or disease, chronic pyelonephritis, amyloidosis

Mechanism/s

Polyuria usually develops via two basic mechanisms: osmotic load and excretion of free water.

1. In some conditions, there is a high 'osmotic load' of the serum being filtered through the kidney due to the *excretion of non-absorbable solutes (e.g. glucose)*. This leads to an *osmotic diuresis*. Put simply, this means large quantities of bigger solutes in the renal tubules of the kidney hold water 'in', rather than allowing it to be reabsorbed. In addition, the concentration gradient in the proximal tubules is altered, affecting sodium reabsorption and urine concentration.

2. The second main pathway is an *inappropriate excretion of free water*,[10] which is usually due to abnormalities in vasopressin production or in response to vasopressin plus an inability to concentrate urine.

Diabetes mellitus

Polyuria in diabetes mellitus is due to *osmotic diuresis* from excretion of excess glucose. The high levels of glucose present exceed the kidney's ability for reabsorption and it is 'lost' in the urine. Water is drawn out by osmosis in the tubule of the kidney. Polyuria in this setting indicates symptomatic hyperglycaemia.

Diabetes insipidus

Diabetes insipidus (DI) can be categorised as either central or peripheral. Nephrogenic DI can be further classified as either congenital or acquired. The basic mechanisms are shown in Table 6.1.

Post-obstructive diuresis

Seen in bilateral urinary tract obstruction, the mechanism behind post-obstructive diuresis/polyuria is complex and is conceptualised in Figure 6.3.

Some research has shown that natriuretic factors[11] such as ANP, which are normally lost in the urine, are retained during the obstructive phase and therefore still exert their effect after the obstruction is relieved. ANP has several actions that facilitate diuresis including blocking the release of renin at the macula densa, blocking the effects of angiotensin 2, and effecting sodium reabsorption and aldosterone release.[12]

TABLE 6.1
Mechanisms of diabetes insipidus (DI)

	Abnormality	Mechanism
Central DI	Idiopathic or secondary to any disorder that leads to damage to the vasopressin (ADH)-secreting neurons in the posterior pituitary	Inadequate excretion of ADH from the pituitary → inadequate activation of the V2 receptors and aquaporins → water is not reabsorbed and is lost in urine
Congenital nephrogenic DI	Mutation of V2 receptor on distal tubule of the kidney	V2 receptor is not responsive to ADH stimulation → failed activation of aquaporin channels → water not appropriately retained and so lost in urine
	Mutation of aquaporin water channel	Mutation of aquaporin water channel does not allow for adequate reuptake of water when the V2 receptor is stimulated by ADH. The water is excreted in urine
Acquired nephrogenic DI	Hypokalaemia	Hypokalaemia leads to decreased expression of aquaporin 2 channels → decreased water uptake and therefore increased diuresis
	Hypercalcaemia	Hypercalcaemia leads to decreased expression of aquaporin 2 channels → decreased water uptake and therefore increased diuresis

Glucose in the urine and drugs for glycaemic control

Knowing the mechanism of reabsorption of glucose in the kidney and the mechanism of polyuria in diabetes helps to understand some of the new therapeutic agents targeting glucose control.

A new class of drugs has been developed to further enhance loss of glucose in the urine to try to improve glycaemic control. The SGLT2 inhibitors inhibit the key sodium–glucose transporter which reabsorbs glucose from the tubules back into the blood. By blocking these, less glucose is reabsorbed; more is lost in the urine and hopefully blood sugar levels fall. Trials have shown reasonable success, with an obvious side effect of mild increase in polyuria.

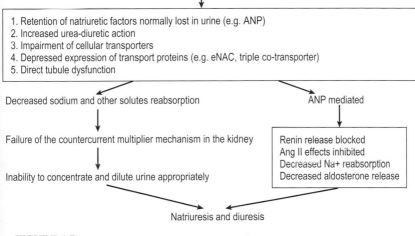

FIGURE 6.3
Mechanisms involved in post–obstructive diuresis

Urinary tract obstruction has also been shown to directly damage tubular function of the kidney and alter the expression of transporter proteins required for the normal handling of solutes and electrolytes. The net result is failure of the countercurrent multiplier mechanism of the kidney, failure of sodium reabsorption and, ultimately, ineffective urinary dilution and concentration. All of these processes contribute to salt and water wasting, resulting in a post-obstructive diuresis.

Lithium

Lithium has a number of effects on the kidney. The relationship between lithium and polyuria is hypothesised to be impairment of the stimulatory effect of ADH on adenylate cyclase[13] which, when present, normally leads to the production of water channels in the cortical collecting duct.

Other influences lithium may have include:

- partial inhibition of aldosterone's capacity to increase eNAC expression and salt reabsorption; as a consequence, salt is lost in the urine and water follows it out[14]

- potentially inhibiting sodium reabsorption in the cortical collecting channel. Decreased sodium reabsorption leads to salt wasting and water follows sodium out in the urine.[15]

References

1. Boccardo P, Remuzzi G, Galbusera M. Platelet dysfunction in renal failure. *Semin Thromb Hemost* 2004;**30**(5):579–89.

2. Mezzano D, Tagle R, Panes O, et al. Hemostatic disorder of uraemia; the platelet defect, main determinant of the prolonged bleeding time, is correlated with indices of activation of coagulation and fibrinolysis. *Thromb Haemost* 1996;**76**:312–21.

3. Sloand EM, Sloand JA, Prodouz K, et al. Reduction of platelet glycoprotein 1B in uraemia. *Br J Haemotol* 1991;**77**:375–81.

4. Fernandez F, Goudable C, Sie P, et al. Low haematocrit and prolonged bleeding time in uraemic patients: effect of red cell transfusions. *Br J Haemotol* 1985;**59**:139–48.

5. Gardner DG, Shoback D. *Greenspan's Basic and Clinical Endocrinology*. 8th ed. New York: McGraw-Hill; 2007.

6. Dunlop D. Eighty-six cases of Addison's disease. *BMJ* 1963;**2**:887.

7. Irvine WJ, Barnes EW. Adrenocortical insufficiency. *Clin Endocrinol Metab* 1972;**1**:549.

8. Klein I, Ojamaa K. Thyroid hormone and the cardiovascular system. *NEJM* 2001; **344**(7):501–9.

9. *Dorland's Medical Dictionary*. 30th ed. Philadelphia: Elsevier; 2003.

10. Walker RJ, Weggery S, Bedford JJ, et al. Lithium-induced reduction in urinary concentrating ability and urinary aquaporin 2 (AQP2) excretion in healthy volunteers. *Kidney Int* 2005;**67**(1):291–4.

11. Harris R, Yarger W. The pathogenesis of post-obstructive diuresis. The role of circulating natriueritc and diuretic factors, including urea. *J Clin Invest* 1975;**56**:880–7.

12. Frokiaer J, Zeidel ML, et al. Chapter 37. Urinary tract obstruction. In: Taal MW, et al., editors. *Brenner and Rector's The Kidney*. 9th ed. Philadelphia: Elsevier; 2011. pp. 1383–410.

13. Garofeanu CG, Weir M, Rosas-Arellano MP, et al. Causes of reversible nephrogenic diabetes insipidus: a systematic review. *Am J Kidney Dis* 2005;**45**(4):626–37.

14. Nielsen J, Kwon TH, Christensen BM, et al. Dysregulation of renal aquaporins and epithelial sodium channel in lithium-induced nephrogenic diabetes insipidus. *Semin Nephrol* 2008;**28**(3):227–44.

15. Bartley GB, Fatourechi V, Kadrmas EF, et al. The incidence of Graves' ophthalmopathy in Olmstead County, Minnesota. *Am J Ophthalmol* 1995; **120**(4):511–17.

6

Figure Credits

Figure 1.1 Based on West JB, *West's Respiratory Physiology*, 7th edn, Philadelphia: Lippincott Williams & Wilkins, 2005: Fig 8-1.

Figure 1.4 Khayat R et al., Sleep-disordered breathing in heart failure: identifying and treating an important but often unrecognized comorbidity in heart failure patients. *Journal of Cardiac Failure* 2013; 19(6): Fig 4. Elsevier 2013.

Figure 1.5 Diaz-Guzman E, Budev MM. Accuracy of the physical examination in evaluating pleural effusion. *Cleveland Clinic Journal of Medicine* 2008; 75(4): 297–303.

Figure 1.7 Based on Aggarwal R, Hunter A, *BMJ*. Available: http://archive.student.bmj.com/issues/07/02/education/52.php [28 Feb 2011].

Figure 1.9 Swartz MH, *Textbook of Physical Diagnosis: History and Examination*, 6th edn, St Louis: Mosby, 2004.

Figure 1.11 Kanchan Ganda, http://ocw.tufts.edu/Content/24/lecturenotes/311144/312054_medium.jpg. © 2006.

Figure 1.14 Based on Manning HL, Schwartzstein RM, *N Engl J Med* 1995; 333(23): 1547–1553.

Figure 1.16 Sun X-G et al., Exercise physiology in patients with primary pulmonary hypertension. *Circulation* 2001; 104: 429–435; Fig 4. AHA 2001.

Figure 1.18 Based on Gardner WN, *Chest* 1996; 109: 516–534.

Figures 1.22, 1.23 Cheng TO, Platypnea-orthodeoxia syndrome: etiology, differential diagnosis and management. *Catheterization and Cardiovascular Interventions* 1999; 47: 64–66.

Figure 2.1 Based on Chatterjee K, Bedside evaluation of the heart: the physical examination. In: Chatterjee K et al. (eds), *Cardiology. An Illustrated Text/Reference*, Philadelphia: JB Lippincott, 1991: Fig 48.5.

Figure 2.2 Based on Vender JS, Clemency MV, Oxygen delivery systems, inhalation therapy, and respiratory care. In: Benumof JL (ed), *Clinical Procedures in Anesthesia and Intensive Care*, Philadelphia: JB Lippincott, 1992: Fig 13-3.

Figure 2.5 Marx JA, Hockberger RS, Walls RM et al. (eds), *Rosen's Emergency Medicine*, 7th edn, Philadelphia: Mosby, 2009: Fig 29.2.

Figure 2.8 Williams RC, Autoimmune disease etiology – a perplexing paradox or a turning leaf? *Autoimmun Rev* 2007-03-01Z, 6(4): 204–208, Fig 2. Copyright © 2006.

Figure 2.9 Douglas G, Nicol F, Robertson C, *Macleod's Clinical Examination*, 13th edn, Churchill Livingstone, Fig 3.6. Copyright © 2013

Figure 2.11 Rangaprasad L et al., Itraconazole associated quadriparesis and edema: a case report. *Journal of Medical Case Reports* 2011; 5: 140.

Figure 2.15 Sack DA, Sack RB, Nair GB, et al., Cholera. *Lancet* 2004; 363: 223–233.

Figures 3.1, 3.2, 3.4 Little JW, Falace DA, Miller CS, Rhodus NL, *Dental Management of the Medically Compromised Patient*, 7th edn, St Louis: Mosby Elsevier, 2008: Figs 25-9, 25-16, 24-6.

Index

Page numbers followed by 'f' indicate figures, 't' indicate tables, and 'b' indicate boxes.